Mehdi Tavassoli
Siamak Ghabeli Zaherkandi
Maryam Milani Fard

Superficial Anatomy and Surgery

Mehdi Tavassoli
Siamak Ghabeli Zaherkandi
Maryam Milani Fard

Superficial Anatomy and Surgery

Upper and Lower Limbs

Noor Publishing

Imprint
Any brand names and product names mentioned in this book are subject to trademark, brand or patent protection and are trademarks or registered trademarks of their respective holders. The use of brand names, product names, common names, trade names, product descriptions etc. even without a particular marking in this work is in no way to be construed to mean that such names may be regarded as unrestricted in respect of trademark and brand protection legislation and could thus be used by anyone.

Cover image: www.ingimage.com

Publisher:
Noor Publishing
is a trademark of
Dodo Books Indian Ocean Ltd., member of the OmniScriptum S.R.L Publishing group
str. A.Russo 15, of. 61, Chisinau-2068, Republic of Moldova Europe
Printed at: see last page
ISBN: 978-620-3-85877-8

Superficial Anatomy and Surgery

Upper and Lower Limbs

By

Dr. Mehdi Tavassoli

Assistant Professor of Orthopaedics, Babol University of Medical Sciences, Iran

Dr. Siamak Ghabeli Zaherkandi

Department of Comparative Anatomy and Embryology, Faculty of Veterinary Medicine, Urmia University, Urmia, Iran

Dr. Maryam Milani Fard

Researcher at the Anesthesia and Pain & Molecular and Cell Biology Research center, Faculty of Medicine Department of Anatomy, Iran University of Medical Sciences, Tehran, Iran
ORCID:0000-0002-0888-8847

Dr. Mehdi Tavassoli

Assistant Professor of Orthopaedics, Babol University of Medical Sciences, Iran

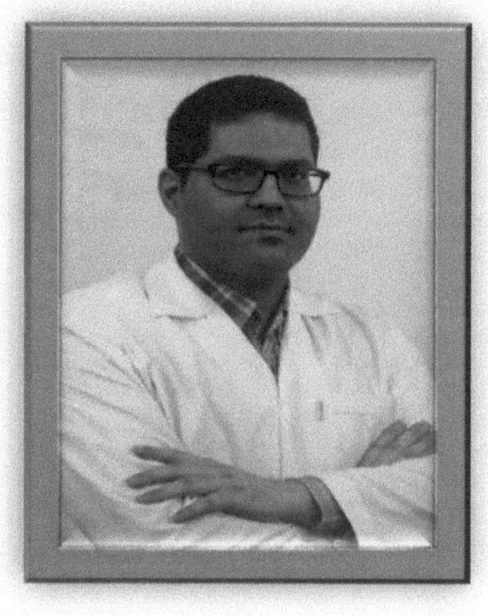

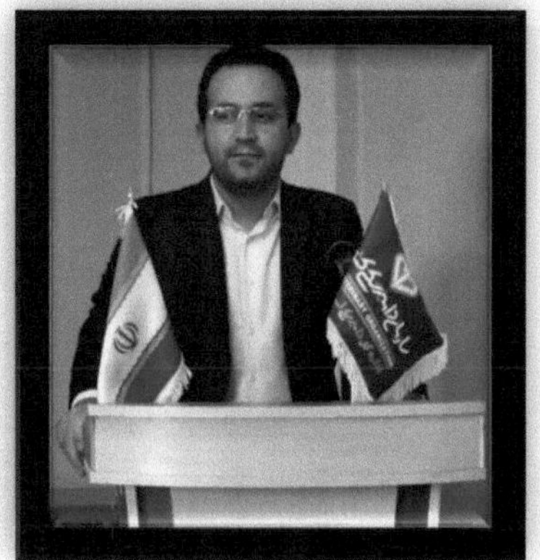

Dr. Siamak Ghabeli Zaherkandi

Department of Comparative Anatomy and Embryology, Faculty of Veterinary Medicine, Urmia University, Urmia, Iran

Dr. Maryam Milani Fard

Researcher at the Anesthesia and Pain & Molecular and Cell Biology Research center, Faculty of Medicine Department of Anatomy, Iran University of Medical Sciences, Tehran, Iran
ORCID:0000-0002-0888-8847

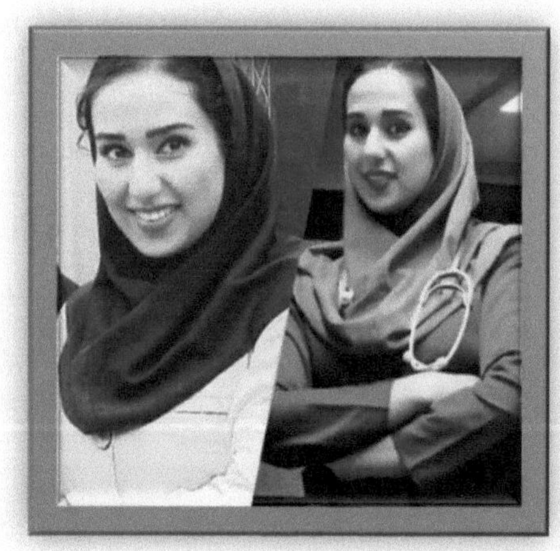

This Book is dedicated to

My Family's

Content

Chapter I

General

Introduction

Anatomy education for medical students is based on corpse dissection in dissection halls, models and museums, although corpse dissection is more relevant to medical students and paramedical students use it less. Learning anatomical structure alone does not have much scientific value, because all examinations and treatments by doctors and paramedics are performed on living people and not on corpses, models, etc. Therefore, the best way to accurately learn the structure of a limb is to study the limb as it naturally exists and functions in the living person. Doctors, surgeons, physiotherapists, nurses, radiologists, artists, etc. should all examine an organ that is covered by skin. Also, examine the function of that organ from under the skin, and this is the responsibility of the superficial anatomy.

Surface anatomy, also called topographic anatomy, is the adaptation of the lower anatomical structures to the surface of the body. A number of structures, such as bony prominences, veins, tendons, and superficial muscles, are easily seen or touched by the skin, which are called landmark signs. We use these signs as well as the actions of those members to examine deeper buildings. Signs are actually our guide to examining buildings and are usually not always visible or prominent, but some depressions or pulses in the arteries are also used as signs. The actions of that member can also be used to examine and observe deeper buildings. For example, to better identify a muscle, we tell the person being examined to contract that muscle.

The study of superficial anatomy should be done on ordinary people, because not all of our patients are athletes (to examine muscles) or thinner (to examine bone points) and so on.

In examining the patient and examining the anatomical structures, you must pay attention to the following points:

1) The patient or model being examined should always and everywhere be considered as a human being. Most people are afraid or guilty of having their body or part of their body exposed. Therefore, it is better to talk to the patient before the examination and give him enough explanations and to minimize the

exposed parts as much as possible. In addition, the patient's religious, ethnic, etc. beliefs must be respected.

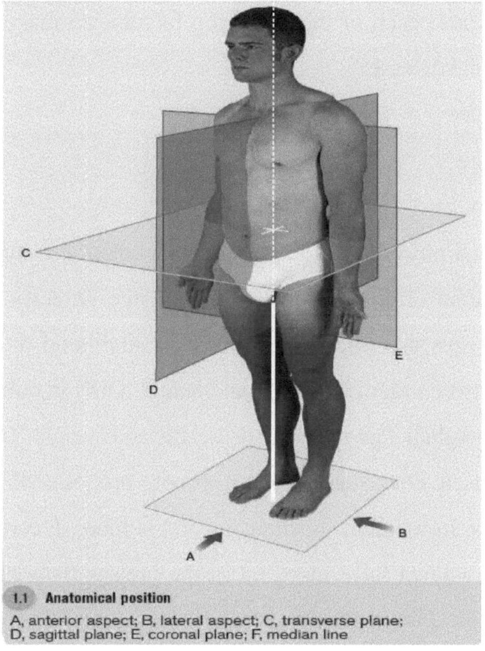

1.1 Anatomical position
A, anterior aspect; B, lateral aspect; C, transverse plane; D, sagittal plane; E, coronal plane; F, median line

Figure 1. Anatomical Position

2) It is necessary to study the superficial anatomy of open eyes, sensitive and precise fingers, calm environment, sufficient light, focused senses, special pencil for marking on the skin and meters. It should be noted that if approximate dimensions such as the width of the hand or fingertip are used, it means the size of the width of the patient's own hand or the person being examined (not the person being examined).
3) The position under study in superficial anatomy is the same as the anatomical position where the person is standing and the upper limbs are hanging on the sides and the palms are facing forward and the thumbs of both feet are placed next to each other.

4) In addition to the items mentioned in the superficial anatomy, the following should always be considered when examining the patient or the person being examined, because each of the following factors can make a difference that is not related to the disease:

A) Race

B) Age

C) sex

Regarding race and physical differences between men and women, it is clear that there are apparent differences that vary with age. In early life, the differences between the sexes are small, and almost to adulthood there are fundamental differences between them in weight and height. Girls in puberty are heavier and taller than boys their age in terms of height and weight. In general, bone and superficial muscle consistency becomes more pronounced with growth in two different sexes. In women, subcutaneous fat is more in certain areas than men. For example, women have more fat in the breasts, buttocks, lower abdomen, thighs and hips. Fat in the lower abdomen causes a slim waist in women compared to men. Fat in men is mostly located in the abdominal wall and mesenteries, and as a result, it causes a bulge in the abdomen or the so-called abdominal corporation.

In men, the symptoms are more pronounced and prominent. The transverse diameter of the upper part of the trunk in the two-shoulder area is larger than the transverse axis in the lower part of the trunk in the pelvic area. While in women, the lower transverse axis is larger than the upper transverse axis. On average, the length of the limbs in women is shorter and shorter than men, and this difference is greater in the lower limbs.

D) Disproportion and symmetry

Lack of proportion and symmetry in any amount can cause changes in the movement and appearance of the member. For example, the shortness of one limb relative to the other, as well as muscle growth and size can be a factor in the development of mismatch in individuals. Like those who do handicrafts, like carpenters and athletes like tennis players, where the difference between right and left hand is often obvious.

E) Physical condition

The structure, shape, and appearance of each person's limbs differ from one person to another, resulting in changes in superficial findings. In terms of physical condition, people can be divided into four groups. This division is mostly related to the trunk and does not include the limbs.

E-1) Hypersthenic (pyknic)

Or bulky physique, wide and short chest and subcostal angle is more open (explosive) so that the heart and lungs are wider and the widest part of the abdomen is located above. The stomach is less longitudinal and the gastric pylorus is relatively high. The transverse colon is really transverse (generally in these people the length and width of the trunk are almost equal).

E-2) Asthenic (Leptosomatic)

These people have a tall and slender body physique and have the following characteristics. Chest long and narrow, angle of closed (acute) subdivisions, longitudinal and narrow heart and lungs, widest part of lower abdomen, longitudinal stomach and relatively low pylorus, V-shaped transverse colon to pelvis may also descend.

E-3) Sthenic

They look more like Hypersthenic.

E-4) Hyposthenic which are more similar to Asthenic.

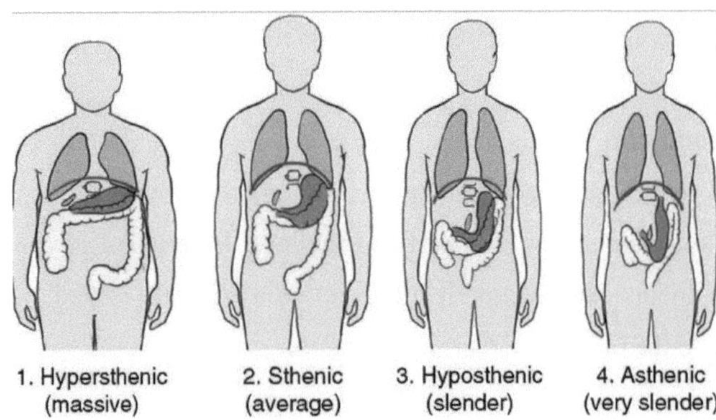

Figure 2. Body mass division

C) Skin

Examination of the body should begin with the skin or mucous membranes. The skin itself plays an important role in the health of the body, and in addition, the skin is almost a full-length mirror inside the body. So the health or disease of the body can be reflected on the skin. The skin and subcutaneous tissues act as a covering for deep structures. But physicians and paramedics must not only be able to locate the organ from the skin, but in certain cases must also evaluate the effectiveness of the organ.

The skin has receptors that inform the body from around it. These receptors are important in parts of the body, such as the palms of the hands. For example, blind people can read the Braille with their fingers, and in these people, the hand also acts as the eye. The characteristics of the skin are different in different parts of the body. This difference is especially noticeable on the lips, which are more prominent than a red skin covered with a thin layer of horns.

Skin appearance: Skin appearance is important to most people because they spend a lot of money and time improving skin quality and appearance. Skin color is due to the presence of melanin pigment in epidermal cells, which is made by melanocytes. The number of melanocytes is not different in different races (black, white, yellow, etc.), but firstly, the amount of melanocyte activity is higher in a person who is darker, and secondly, melanin is present in different people in different colors from yellow to brown or black. Ultraviolet light increases the activity of melanocytes.

Attachment of the skin to the underlying tissue: As the skin should be attached to the underlying tissue, this adhesion should not be such as to prevent the free movement of the underlying structures (such as muscles). With age, the elasticity of the skin decreases and the skin becomes wrinkled. For example, if you hold the skin on the back of young people with two fingers and lift it up and then release it, the skin will return to its original state almost immediately, but in older people this return will be much later. In certain areas, such as the skin folds of the palm, the skin must adhere to the deep fascia below so that it can move freely without the tissues being squeezed between the skin and the fat under the skin.

The skin adjusts the contour of the body regardless of movement, although this is due to the intrinsic elasticity of the skin and its calculated connection. However, in some places the skin is exposed to internal pressures that vary in different areas. Langer showed that even in corpses, the skin is exposed to pressures in certain directions. He drew these lines.

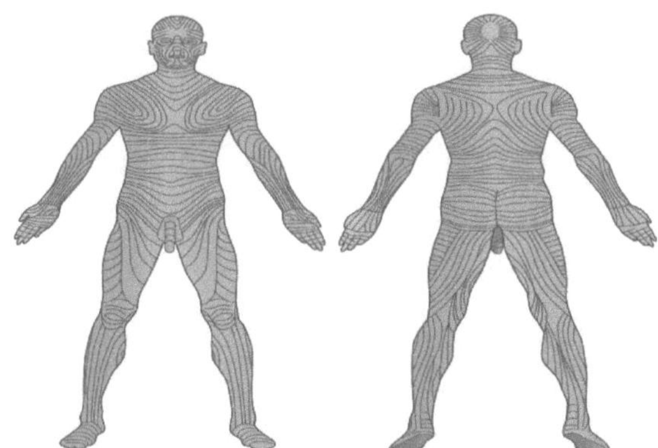

Figure 3. Anterior and posterior view of cutaneous dermatomes

These lines are due to the arrangement of collagen fibers in the skin (Derm) and are more commonly known as Langer's lines. If surgical incisions are made in the direction of these lines, the wound will heal with minimal scarring. Langer lines do not always match the pressure lines in life. Therefore, it may be better to consider these lines as resting stress lines.

Langer's Lines

In addition to the resting pressure lines, creases are seen on parts of the skin that are due to the skin adhering to the underlying connective tissue (such as the skin adhering to the palmar aponeurosis) or flexion or extension folds. creases) (such as folds behind the knee or groin). In certain areas, such as the face, neck, and palms, the peripheral muscles attach directly to the skin, producing movement in the skin. As a result, these muscles can create dynamic stress lines in addition to resting pressure lines. In some places, smooth muscles contract in response to stimuli (cold, etc.) and create wrinkles in the skin (such as the skin of the testicles and the skin around the areola).

D) Hair

The skin of all parts of the body except the palms and soles of the feet and lips is covered by hair to varying degrees. In many areas and individuals, especially women and children, hair may be fine and fuzzy. But in other areas in men, the hair may be very clear and coarse. In many areas of the body, the hair has a direction. In addition, the hair is controlled by fine smooth muscles that straighten in cold weather or fear. In the scalp, hair has major differences in color and structure. Some men may develop baldness, which does not indicate a specific pathology, but baldness in women usually indicates a pathological aspect.

H) Bones

Most of the appearance of the body surface is caused by the skeletal and muscular skeletons attached to them. From the axial skeleton, the skull, part of the teeth and vertebrae are easily touched. The pelvis is mostly covered by muscles, but some parts are prominent. In the limbs, some parts of the bone are hidden by the muscles, but some parts can be used as anatomical signs.

F) Muscles

Some muscles are covered by skin and fascia and even fat, but some muscles are obvious even in non-muscular people. Few people can contract a specific muscle on their own. Therefore, the examiner should instruct the patient to make movements that involve contraction of the target muscle. It should be noted that under normal circumstances, muscles do not work alone but work in groups. In fact, even when the body is at rest, all the muscles of the body contribute to this state of rest and show a small amount of action potential. Because even in professional athletes, gymnasts, etc., it is impossible to move most of the muscles alone, in order to examine the muscles for their specific action and therefore the normality of their nervousness, attention should be paid to the movement of a group of muscles.

Usually, if the movement of the muscle is not easily defined from the surface, it is necessary to compare the muscle of one side with the other (of course, one should also consider the strength of one side due to the job).

When examining muscles, keep in mind that some muscles only pass through one joint and act on that joint, while others pass over more than one joint and therefore work on several joints. Flexor digitorum longus flexors theoretically work on several joints. Therefore, the effect will be on an insufficient joint. Muscles cannot exert their maximum strength on more than one joint. So multijoints will naturally work with other muscles or sometimes with ligaments to fix the rest of the joints and the muscle will only work on one joint. When the long flexor muscles of the fingers contract, the fingers cannot work effectively unless the wrist and midcarpal joints are fixed. Conversely, if the wrist is not fixed, the fingers will bend poorly, so the examiner will notice a defect in the flexor muscle, which is not the case.

Multi-joint muscles may not be able to contract or stretch enough to move all the joints that pass through them. For example, the hamstrings pass over the hip and knee joints, extending the hip joint and flexing the knee joint. But if the hip joint is open, the bending power of their knee joint decreases and the knee cannot bend completely. This condition is called active insufficiency. Active muscle inadequacy can be demonstrated by taking a knife from an attacker. If the wrist is straight, the knife is held firmly in the hand, but when the wrist is bent, the knife is lost.

If the action of a muscle on a joint is stopped or weakened by muscles working in the opposite direction on the same joint, it is called passive insufficiency. For example, if a person has a bent knee, he can bend his hip joint to about 115-120 degrees. But when the person's knee is straight (due to the opposite muscles behind the thigh and opening the hip joint), the bending of the hip joint reaches about 60-80 degrees. In short, in the active type, a part of the muscle itself prevents its activity, but in the inactive type, the muscle will prevent its activity by acting against it (Agonist).

G) Proportions of the body

The proportions of different parts of the body change greatly with age. The nervous system must be almost completely formed before birth. So the nerve tissue of the brain, spinal cord, and peripheral nerves is actually complete at birth.

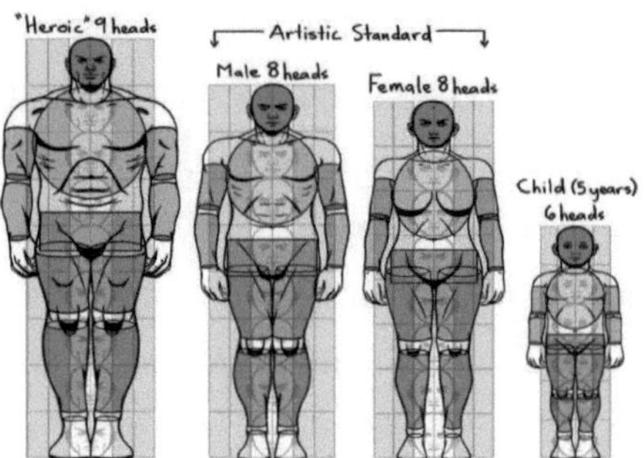

Figure 4. Body changes with age

The growth of nerve fibers and myelination will continue until 1.5-2 years of age, at which time the cranial cavity reaches its maturity, and from now on there are more bone changes, especially in the face. Meanwhile, the trunk and some more organs grow and thus change the proportions of the body. Different body proportions and sizes are:

1. While in the adult the eyes are in the middle of the height of the head, in the infant the eyes are closer to the chin and the ratio of the eyes up and down is two thirds.
2. In an adult, the head has between one-seventh and one-eighth the total height of the body (13%), while at birth this ratio is one-fourth and at two years of age one-fifth.
3. The midpoint of adult height is in the pubic symphysis, while this point is in the baby in the umbilicus or above it. Therefore, the length of the lower limbs of an adult is equal to half his height, but in the baby, it will be about one third of his height.
4. The size of the upper limb from the shoulder to the fingertips in an adult is two-fifths of his height, but in infants this ratio is higher.
5. If an adult open both hands completely and the hand is 90 degrees away from his body, the distance between the two middle fingers of the hand will be equal to his height.
6. The length of an adult when kneeling is equal to the length of the same person up to the axilla (standing) axillary position. In other words, the length of the lower limb from the knee down is equal to the distance from the armpit to the top of the head.
7. The sitting height of each person is a little more than half of his standing height.

   It should be noted that the face ratios will be entered in the relevant section.

Note: The following formula is used to determine the approximate body surface (Body surface) of a person:

(90 + body weight in kilograms) {{+7 (4 body weight in kilograms)} = total body surface area in square meters

Rule 9 (Rule of Nine) can be used to gain the level of approximately any part of the body. This rule is mostly used to determine the percentage of body surface burns. This rule divides the body into 11 regions of 9% and the remaining one percent is related to the external genitalia. The other areas are:

- Head 9%
- Upper limbs 9% each
- 9% front of each lower limb
- 9% behind each lower limb
- 9% front chest
- Back of the chest 9%
- 9% anterior abdomen
- Back of the abdomen 9%

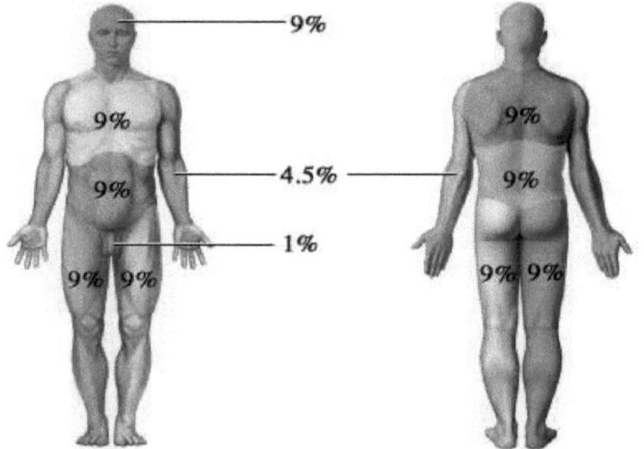

Figure 5. Percentage of different areas of the body

Chapter II

Superficial Anatomy of the Upper Limb

The lower limbs are articulated with the pelvis, but the upper limbs are designed to work with maximum control from the trunk. Therefore, the movement between the lower limb and the trunk is limited to the spherical joint of the thigh, however, in the case of the upper limb, there is considerable movement between the shoulder girdle and the trunk and within the joint itself. In this chapter, first the signs of bones and joints, then muscles and tendons, cavities, grooves and depressions, and finally the path of nerves, arteries, veins and lymph will be examined.

Bone points of the upper limb

Clavicle

It is S-shaped and can be felt under the skin along its entire length. The inner part of the bone is convex to the front and the arteries and nerves of the upper limb pass through it from the back, while the outer part is concave to the front. Due to the protrusion of the inner end of the two clavicles, the jugular notch deepens the sternum. When the arm is abducted, the outer end of the clavicle and acromion is placed inside a depression formed by the deltoid muscle. In females, the clavicle is shorter, thinner, arched, and smoother, with the acromial end at a lower level than the outer end, while in males the two ends are at the same level or the outer end is slightly Is placed higher.

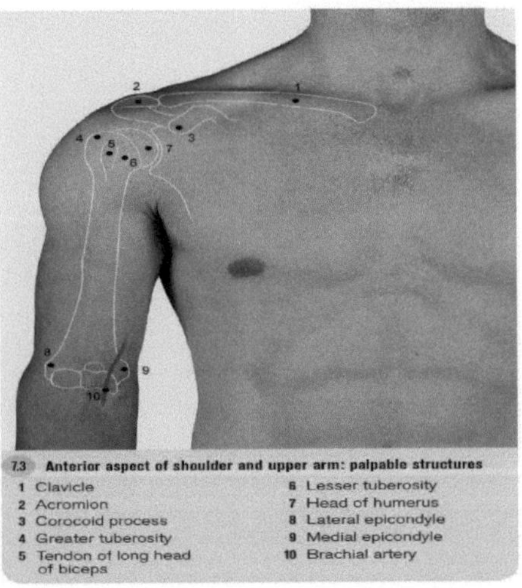

Figure 6. Anterior view of superficial shoulder anatomy

Scapula

The bone is triangular and wide, located between the second and seventh ribs. Many muscles attach to it and actually act as a support for the muscles. However, parts of the bone are palpable or visible and are used as a landmark in superficial anatomy.

Spine

The side of the back of the thorn, called the crest, is completely under the skin and is easy to touch. In thin people it is a prominent line, but in muscular people it is palpable between the upper and lower muscle masses. The outer end of the spine continues as the acromion, and the inner end, when the arm is placed on the side, is at the level of the thorny appendage of the third vertebra (T_3) or the body of the fourth vertebra (T_4). This end is also adjacent to the fourth gear. At the lower edge of the spine, about 2.5 cm from the inner end, is the deltoid tubercle, which is sometimes touched. To touch the scapula, it is better to turn the hand inwards, in this case, the spike becomes horizontal and palpable.

Acromion (last addition)

The outer end is the scapula and is clearly seen in some people. That is why it is called the Point of shoulder. The intersection of the outer and posterior edges of the acromion is called the acromial angle or apex and can be detected by precise touch. This point is used as a fixed point to measure the length of the upper limb and compare the two limbs. The clavicle, acromion, and scapula together form a bony arch, which is the best position to observe and examine this arch.

Coracoid process

On the outside of the cavity below the clavicle (Infraclavicular fossa) is approximately 2.5 cm below the junction of the outer quarter and the rest of the clavicle. To touch it, you have to push up and out in the depth of the deltoid muscle, or place the palms of both hands on the deltoid muscle in two directions and touch this appendage with two thumbs in the cavity below the clavicle and the margin of the deltoid muscle. It can sometimes be mistaken for a small humerus (Lesser tubercle). For differential diagnosis, it is enough to rotate the shoulder joint. If rotation does not occur, it is related to the coracoid appendage.

Inferior angle

Although it is covered by muscles, it is perfectly defined and is located in a standing position on the seventh rib or seventh space between the teeth and on the level of the thorn of the seventh vertebra (T_7) and the body of the eighth vertebra (T_8). In the various movements that occur in the shoulder, you can usually see the lower angle. The lower angle is used as a marker to count the ribs and examine the patient. The top angle is on the second gear and is palpable because it is covered by muscles.

Medial border

It is pulled from the second to the seventh gear. The serratus anterior muscle causes the scapula and its inner side to attach to the chest, and when this muscle is active, the inner side is not clear. But when this muscle is at rest, it becomes clear and palpable. When this muscle is paralyzed, the inside of the scapula becomes too prominent, creating a wing-like position on the back (Winging of the scapula). The outer side of the scapula is not easily touched except at the bottom.

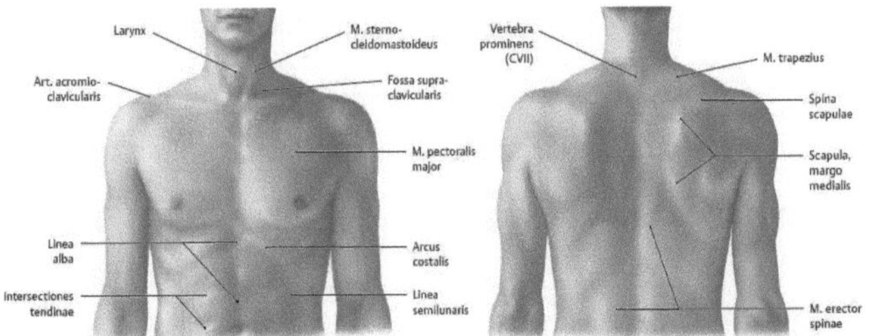

Figure 7. Anterior superficial anatomy and posterior trunk

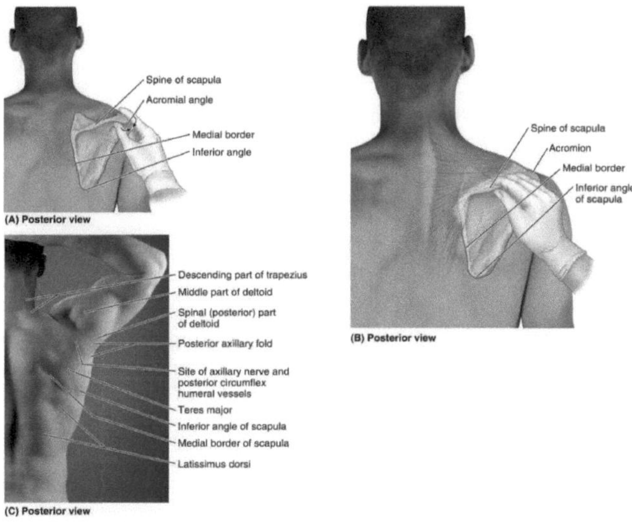

Figure 8. Superficial anatomy of the scapula and back

Humerus

Its tangible parts are:

Greater tubercle: It forms the outermost point of the bone in the shoulder area. It is located immediately below the acromion appendage, and by turning the arm inward and outward, this bulge is felt on the outer front. Of course, this bulge is covered by the deltoid muscle. This bulge, along with the deltoid muscle, causes the shoulder to round, and in the sound of deltoid paralysis or dislocation of the shoulder joint, the shoulder roundness disappears and the acromion becomes prominent.

Lesser tubercle: It is covered by the deltoid, but by deep pressure and turning the arm inwards, it can be touched about 3 cm below the acromion appendage below and outside the coracoid appendage.

Head: By rotating in and out of the shoulder joint, it can be touched to the floor of the axilla.

Surgical neck: It is covered by the deltoid muscle and is surrounded by the axillary nerve and the circumflex arteries of the arm. The surgical neck is located about 5 cm below the acromial appendage. The surgical neck can be felt on the outer surface of the axilla next to the Coracobrachialis muscle.

Body: It is mostly covered by muscles but can be easily touched.

Deltiod tuberosity: Below the adhesion of the deltoid muscle on the outer surface of the arm is palpable.

Medial epicondyle: Because the flexors attach to it, it is also called the flexor epicondyle. This relatively large subcutaneous bulge is easily palpable on the inside of the elbow and behind it is a groove through which the ulnar nerve passes, and pressure on it, especially in thin people, may make the nerve feel pressure or uncomfortable. This is why this part of the bone is called the funny bone.

Lateral epicondyle: It is smaller than the internal epicondyle. When the elbow is open (Extended), there is a depression in the outer back of the elbow that can be felt in the depth of this external epicondyle depression.

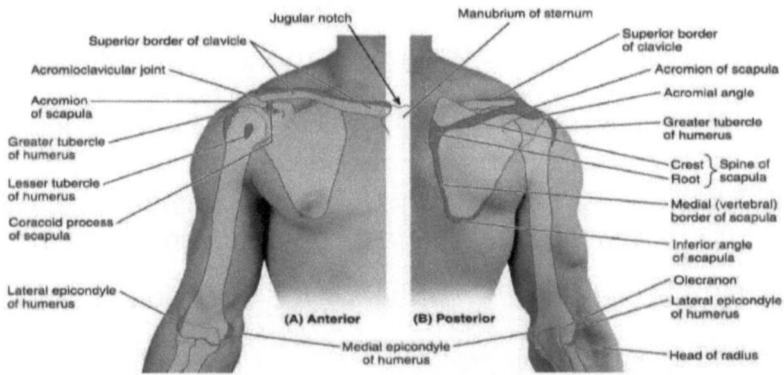

Figure 9. Superficial anatomy of the bones of the upper limbs and trunk

Ulna bone: The palpable parts of the ulna are

Elbow appendage (Olecranon): The highest part of the bone is the ulna and in the open elbow it can be touched on the line that connects the two epicondyles of the arm, but when the elbow is bent, the upper end of this appendage is lowered and at the same time with the two epicondyles of the arm an equal triangle They create sides. This condition changes in fractures around the joint.

Posterior border: It is thick, round and subcutaneous, and when the elbow is bent, it is located below the longitudinal groove behind the forearm and between two muscular ridges. This side may be touched up to the ulna of the ulna (styloid process).

Head: The inner surface of the back of the wrist can be seen and touched when it is in the pronation position.

Styloid process

When the palm is facing up (Supination), this growth may be felt just below the bone head and on the inside of the Extensor carpi ulnaris muscle tendon.

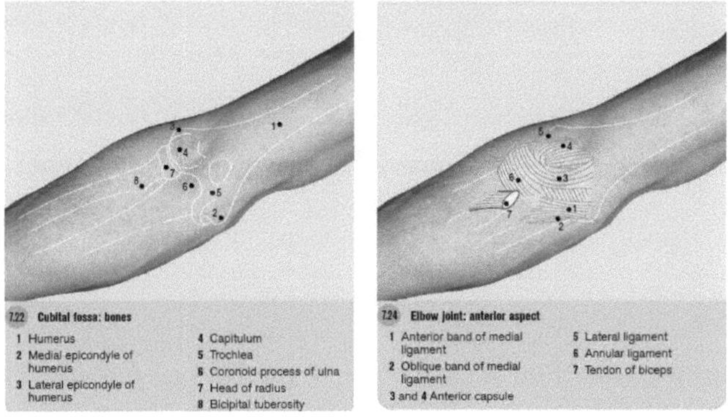

Figure 10. Superficial anatomy and elbow joint surgery

Radius bone

Tangible signs include:

Head Radius: When the elbow is fully open, touch the outside of the back of the elbow below the external epicondyle. If the two index and middle fingers are stuck together in the hollow of the outer part behind the elbow and the upper finger is on the outer epicondyle, the lower finger will represent the head of the radius. By rotating in and out of the forearm, the radius head and even the joint space between the radius head and the humerus can be easily touched.

Radial styloid process

Anatomical snuff box can be touched on the upper part of the floor. To touch it, it is better to put the hand in the pronation position. This angle is about one centimeter lower than the appendage of the ulna bone. This is important for surgeons in the treatment of Colle's fracture of the lower extremity.

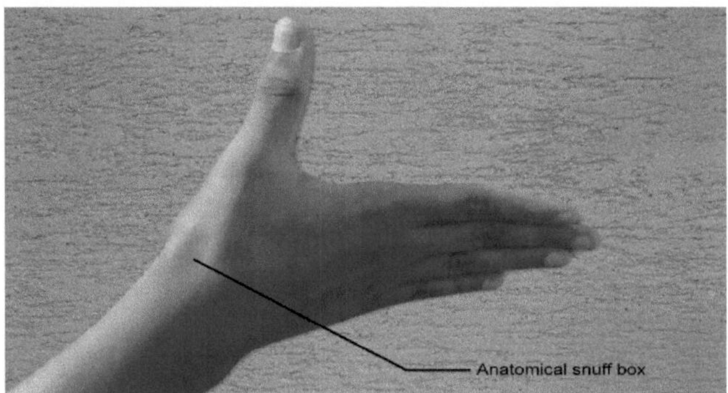

Figure 11. Superficial anatomical anatomy of the snuff box

Lateral border

It can be felt in the middle third of the forearm. Also, the outer surface is easily touched in the lower half of the radius. In addition, the front, outer, and dorsal surfaces of the lower end of the radius, which are covered by tendons, are palpable.

Dorsal or Lister tubercle of radius

If the wrist is bent forward, the bulge is felt on the dorsal surface of the lower end of the radius. This protrusion is also the surface of the ulna's head, and if you pull upwards from the space between the index and middle fingers on the back of the handwriting, you will reach it.

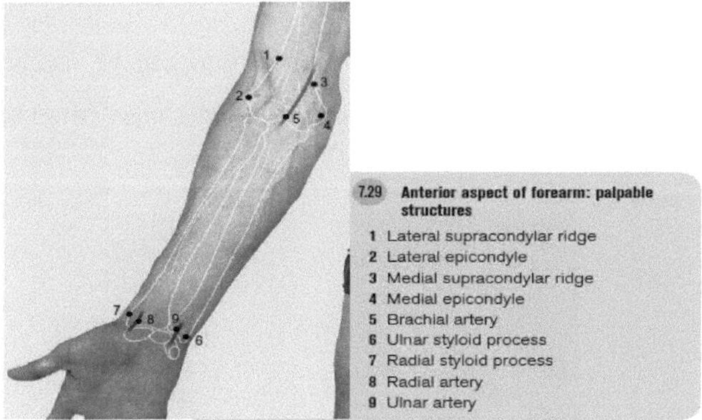

Figure 12. Superficial anatomy of the anterior forearm

Bone points of wrist and hand

Scaphoid

The bone itself is felt below the radius of the radius in the anatomical ventricle, but its tubercle is located on the anterior surface of the bone. The Flexor carpi radialis tendon is identified. Especially when the hand is bent outwards (Radial deviation = abduction). To find the tubercle, you can also pull up the line from the middle finger to reach the crease of the wrist. This bone breaks more than any other wrist bone.

Tubercle of trapezium

It can be felt about one centimeter below the scaphoid tubercle and slightly outside with deep pressure.

Pea bone (Pisifrom)

Right in front of the inner end of the distal crease, the wrist is touched in the inner part of the upper side of the hypothenar ridge, and if you continue the Flexor carpi ulnaris tendon towards the distal, you will reach this bone.

Hook of hamate

About one centimeter below the pea bone (Pisifrom) can be touched with deep pressure. If you draw a line from the outside of the fourth finger (ring) to the pisiform bone, the hook is on this line.

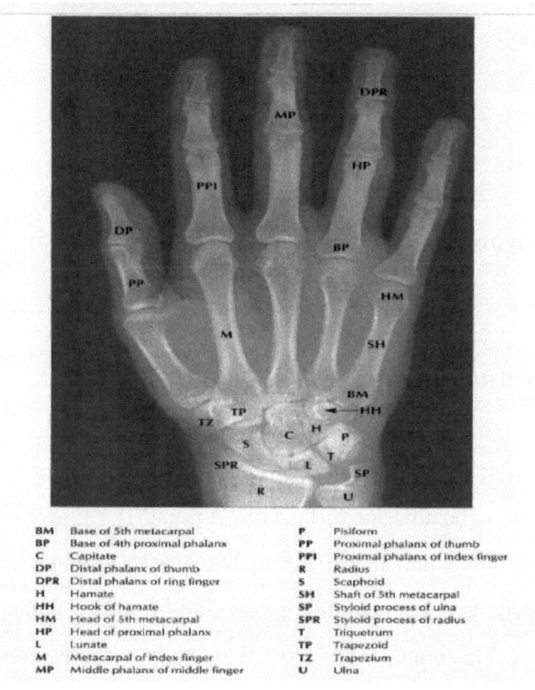

Figure 13. Radiology view of hands and fingers

Crescent (Lunate)

If the wrist is bent, it can be felt in the space between the two protrusions of the radius and ulna. This bone dislocation is more common than all wrist bones.

Capital

Slightly above the base of the third metacarp, there is a shallow depression in the back of the hand, located deep inside the bone.

Metacarpals and Phalanges

They are easily touched, especially from the back surface. When the hand is punched, the metacarpal heads are visible along with their protrusions, called knuckle prominence.

Joints of upper limb

Sternoclavicular joint

It is the only joint between the upper limb and the trunk, and this connection is not very strong. This joint does not bear much weight and the joint cavity is divided into two parts by a fibrocartilage disc. In this joint, unlike other joints in the body that have clear cartilage, it is fibrous cartilage. This joint is located between the two ends of the Sternocleidomastoid muscle (SCM). By raising and lowering the shoulder, the joint depression will be palpable. This joint is very important in terms of superficial anatomy, because it is used as an important landmark on the head, neck, trunk and upper limbs.

Acromioclavicular joint

If you move about 3 cm from the top of the acromion angle along the outer side of the acromion, this joint and the outer end of the clavicle will be touched.

Shoulder joint

To determine the boundaries of the shoulder joint, first find the coracoid appendage, then attach it to the acromion appendage. Then draw a vertical line from the middle of the inner third (near the coracoid process) at a distance of 1.5-2 cm. In this way, the shoulder joint is obtained from the front.

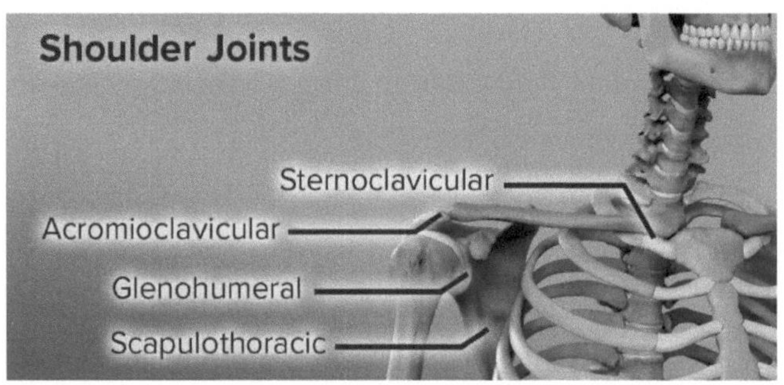

Figure 14. Shoulder belt

Elbow joint

In the case where the elbow is open, if the two epicondyles of the humerus are connected by a line, the joint line is identified.

Carrying cubital angle

Because the inside of the trochlea is about 6 mm or less from the Capitulum, and because of the inclination of the upper articular surface of the coronoid, when the elbow is fully extended and the forearm is outstretched (supination), the forearm bones are slightly They are bent outwards and the inner side of the arm is not along the inner side of the forearm, and the forearm deviates 5-5 degrees from the inner side of the arm to the outside, which is called the carrying angle (although in some sources The outer side of the arm and the outer side of the forearm, which is between 160-175 degrees, are considered). This angle prevents the hands and objects from colliding with the body when carrying objects, and due to the fact that the pelvis is wider in women, this angle is more in women. This angle disappears when the elbow is bent due to the equal joint surfaces of the humerus and ulna. This angle depends on height, weight, age and physical activity. So that with age, this angle also increases and is also less in athletes. If this angle is greater than usual, it is called Cubitus valgus. It should be noted that in fact we mostly carry objects between Suspination and Pronation forearm.

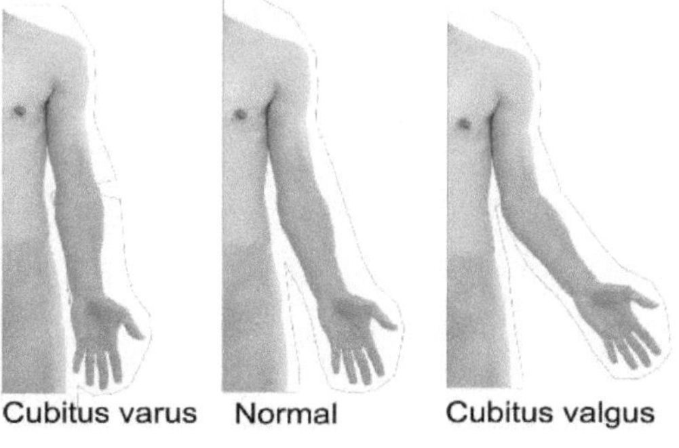

Figure 15. Abnormality of carrying Angle

Wrist or Radiocarpal joint: If you connect the base of the ulna and radius styloid appendages, the wrist joint line becomes clear, which is not completely horizontal due to the slightly lower radius styloid appendage.

Muscles and tendons of the upper limb

Shoulder muscles

Too many muscles in the shoulder area are superficial and deep that act on the shoulder girdle or shoulder joint. Some of these muscles are visible and palpable, but others are directly palpable and visible, and their operation can indicate that they are healthy or sick. A muscle is better defined when it contracts, and it is better to resist what the muscle is doing. For example, to observe and touch the biceps brachii, you should ask your friend to bend his elbow and resist the action by applying force in the opposite direction. In other words, try to open your friend's elbow. In this case, the biceps muscle or tendon is more clearly seen or touched. The muscles of the shoulder area that can be felt and seen are:

Pectoralis major: It is in the form of a fan and can be seen and touched. The resistance of the whole muscle is determined by the resistance to adduction. If the arm moves obliquely upwards and towards the head and there is resistance to its movement, the fibers of the upper part (Clavicular) are separated and when the arm approaches the body in the lower position, the lower part (Sternocotalis) contracts turns. The lower side of the muscle forms the anterior axillary fold. There is a Deltopectoral groove between the upper part and the deltoid muscle. The upper part of this groove is along the cavity below the clavicle (Infraclavicular fossa). The cephalic vein and deltoid artery pass through this groove.

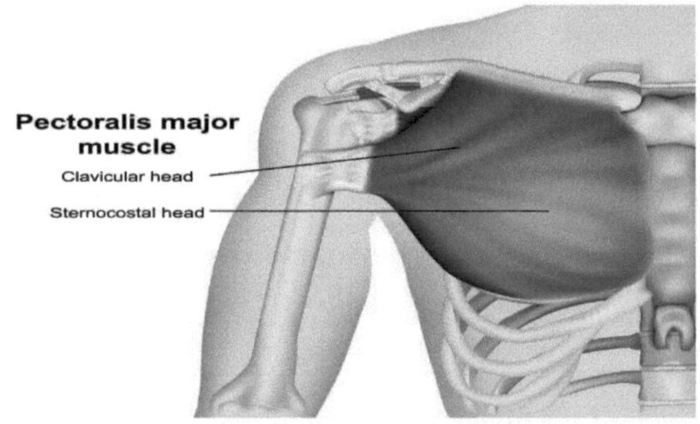

Figure 16. Superficial anatomy of the pectoralis major muscle

Pectoralis minor: Completely covered by Pectoralis major. To touch this muscle, place the forearm in the lower back. Because the pectoralis major muscle is at rest, the small thoracic tendon can be felt just below the Coracoid process. This muscle can also be felt on the back of the front wall of the axilla.

Serratus anterior (front teeth): To determine this, ask the patient to place his hands on the wall and apply force to the front (when pushing the car). Also, when the arm is placed above the head, the lower bands of the muscle near their connection to the ribs may be seen and touched.

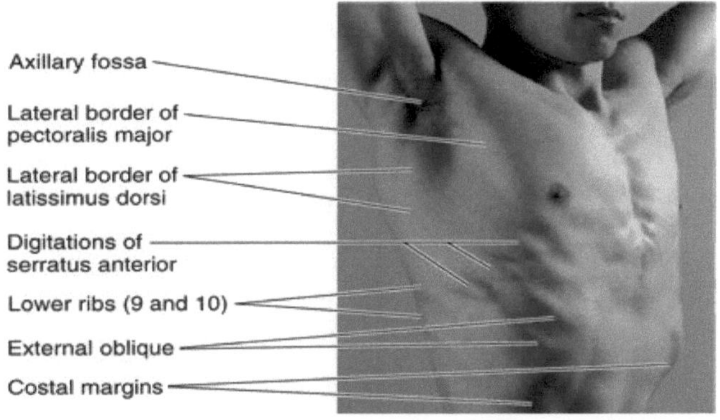

Figure 17. Superficial anatomy of the anterior view of the trunk

Deltoid (Dolly Shape)

It has three parts: front, middle and back. While the elbow is open, all parts of the muscle are characterized by resistance to abduction. At the lower end is the palpable deltoid tuberosity. This muscle is used for intramuscular injections with low fluid content (such as insulin).

Trapezius or Schawl muscle

Anatomists first called it the Cucullaris muscle. To mark its parts, the person raises his arms above the level of the horizon (Adduction) and at the same time moves the shoulder belt backwards (Retraction). The anterior side participates in the formation of the dorsal triangle of the neck and the supraclavicular fossa.

Supraspinatus (above the thorn)

When the elbow is open and the forearm is in the midpronation position and the arm is on the side, start abducting the arm. This muscle is felt below the Trapezius muscle. The action of this muscle is to start abduction of the arm up to an angle of 30 degrees. If this muscle is paralyzed, the operation to move the arm away from the body should initially be carried by the other hand up to 30 degrees, or the person should bend towards the paralyzed muscle so that the hand is about 30 degrees away from the body.

The deltoid is responsible for moving the arm more than 30 degrees from the body to the horizon, and from there it is responsible for the Serratus Anterior and Trapezius.

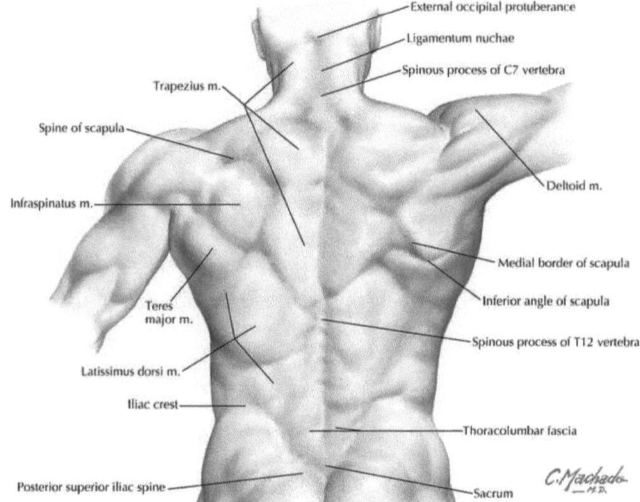

Figure 18. Superficial anatomy of the posterior view of the trunk

Teres minor and infra spinatus

With the elbow bent 90 degrees and the arm 90 degrees away from the body, rotate the shoulder joint outward and resist rotation. In this case, the fibers of these two muscles are identified. In some people, these two muscles are not recognizable.

Teres major

The underside is smaller and larger than that. If there is resistance to bringing the arm closer to the trunk (adduction), the muscle is touched outside the lower angle of the scapula.

Latissmus dorsi (dorsal area)

If there is resistance to bringing the arm closer to the trunk (Adduction) and pulling it back (Extension), this muscle will contract along with the large round. These two muscles together form the posterior axillary fold.

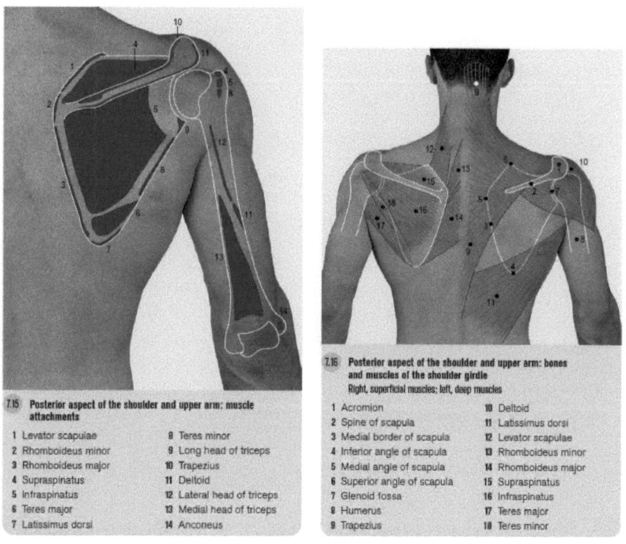

Figure 19. Superficial anatomy and surgery of the bones and muscles of the back

Arm muscles

Biceps brachii (double arm)

By applying resistance to bending the elbow, the muscle and even the two heads and tendons are identified. In order to observe and touch its forearm (Bicipital aponeurosis) in the same position, the forearm must be turned against resistance (Supination). Its tendon and nipple are located in the elbow cavity. On the inside and outside of this muscle are two internal and external gutters in the arm area known as medial and lateral bicipital grooves. In the external gutter, which is wide and indistinct, a cephalic vein is placed. The inner groove joins the axillary cavity at the top. These two grooves reach the elbow cavity (Cubital fossa) at the bottom. Some authors also call the medial and lateral cubital fossa by the same name. Intertubercular groove in the humerus is also known as Bicipital groove.

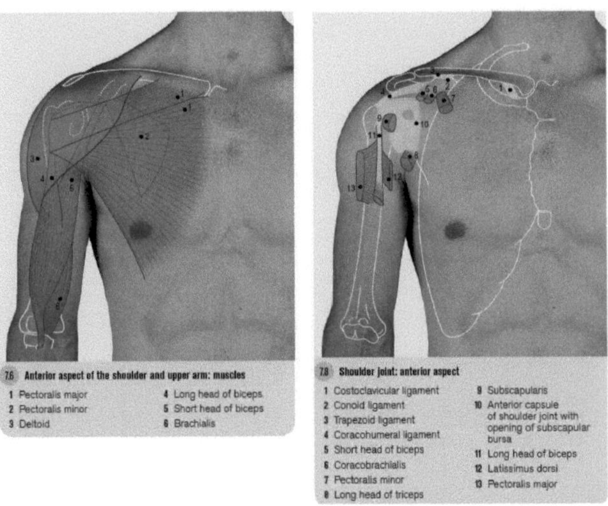

Figure 20. Superficial anatomy and surgery of bones and anterior muscles

Coracobrachialis

The upper bouts featured two cutaways, for easier access to the higher frets. The lower bouts featured two cutaways, for easier access to the higher frets.

Brachialis (arm)

When the forearm is turned inward (Pronation) and the elbow is bent because the biceps muscle relaxes, this muscle is touched.

Triceps brachii (three arms)

With resistance to opening the elbow (Extemsion) is well defined in the back of the arm. The long head is visible from under the lower fibers of the dorsal part of the deltoid, and the outer head of the muscle is slightly lower than the dorsal part of the deltoid. The inner head is covered in part by its long head and the lower part is palpable near the inner epicondyle of the arm.

Forearm muscles

Brachioradialis

When the forearm is in midpronation position, it is well defined by its resistance to flexion of the elbow on the outside of the forearm.

Pronator teres

While the arm is on the side and the elbow is bent about 135 degrees, it is touched obliquely by resisting rotation into the forearm (pronation) and bending the elbow further at the top of the forearm.

Flexor carpi radialis

When resistance is established against abduction and flexion of the wrist, it is the first tendon to be identified on the outside of the wrist, and it can be seen that the muscle tendon passes over the scaphoid bone. Between this tendon and the Brachioradialis muscle tendon is the pulse groove, and the pulse of the radial artery can be felt in the wrist.

Palmaris longus

It may not be present in some people, but if it is present, it is characterized by resistance to wrist flexion. A better way to see this tendon is to bring the thumb closer to the little finger (Opposition). This tendon is used for tendon grafting. The tendon is located between the tendon and the Flexor carpi radialis tendon in the wrist of the median nerve.

Flexor digitorum superficialis

By punching and resisting flexion of the wrist, the muscle tendons can be felt immediately above the wrists and inside the Palmaris longus tendon. In addition, when there is no Palmaris longus muscle, the tendons of this muscle are much better identified. Especially the tendon that points to the finger and may be confused with the Palmaris longus tendon.

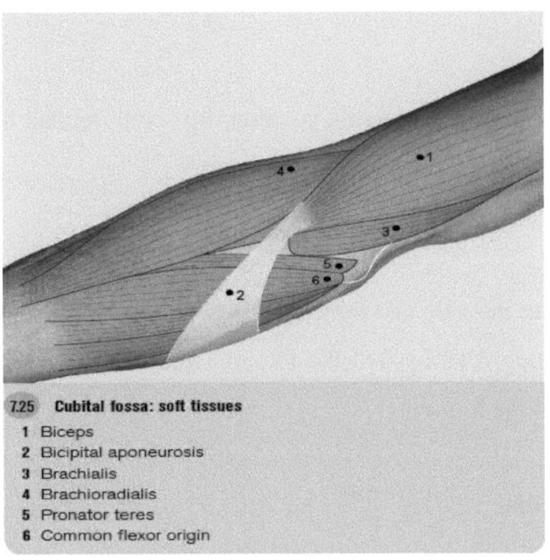

Figure 21. Superficial anatomy and elbow and forearm surgery

Flexor carpi ulnaris

When the forearm is complete in supination and the fingers are loose, with flexion of the wrist and its bending inwards (Adduction), the muscle tendon is determined and by following the tendon, we reach the Pisiform bone. Also, by punching the hand, the muscle tendon is observed and touched in the innermost part of the wrist, immediately outside the tendon in the wrist, the nerve and the ulnar artery are located.

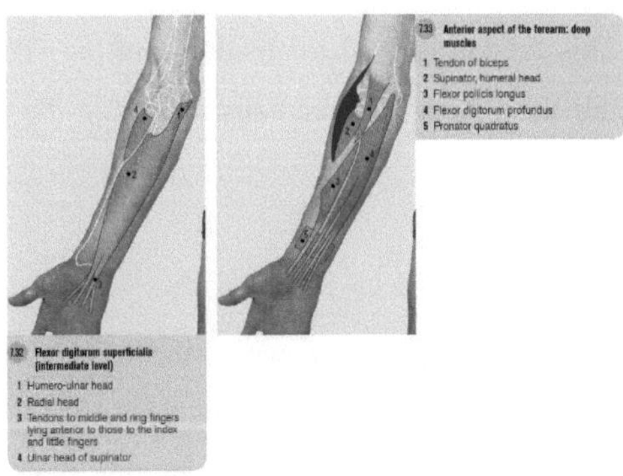

Figure 22. Superficial anatomy and elbow and forearm surgery

To determine the direction of the superficial muscles in the front of the forearm, the heel of one hand can be placed on the inner epicondyle of the other hand. In this case, the five fingers represent the five superficial muscles of the front of the forearm in the following order from outside to inside:

1) thumb = Pronator teres

2) Finger = Flexor carpi radialis

3) Middle finger = Palmaris longus

4) Finger ring = Flexor digitorum superficialis

5) Little finger = Flexor carpi ulnaris

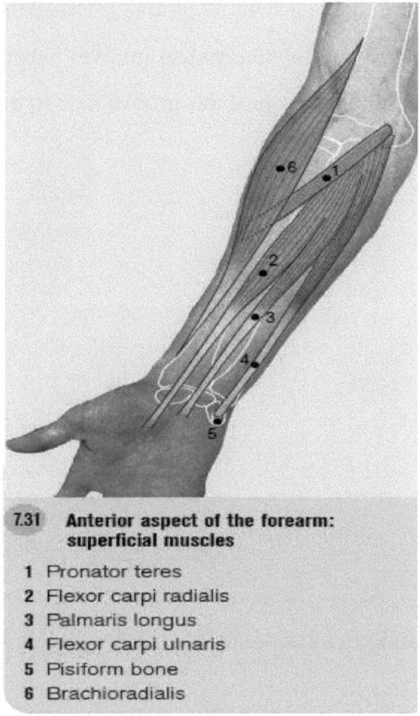

Figure 23. Superficial anatomy and forearm surgery

Muscles behind the forearm

By tapping and pressing the waist or bending the elbow and resisting the opening of the wrist above the forearm from the outside to the inside, the following muscles are partially identified:

1) Brachioradialis

2) Extensor carpi radialis longus

3) Extensor carpi radialis brevis

4) Extensor digitorum

5) Extensor carpi ulnaris There is a shallow groove between the last two muscles.

6) Flexor carpi ulnaris There are relatively clear grooves between the muscles number 5 and 6, which can be felt in the depth of this groove next to the back of the ulna.

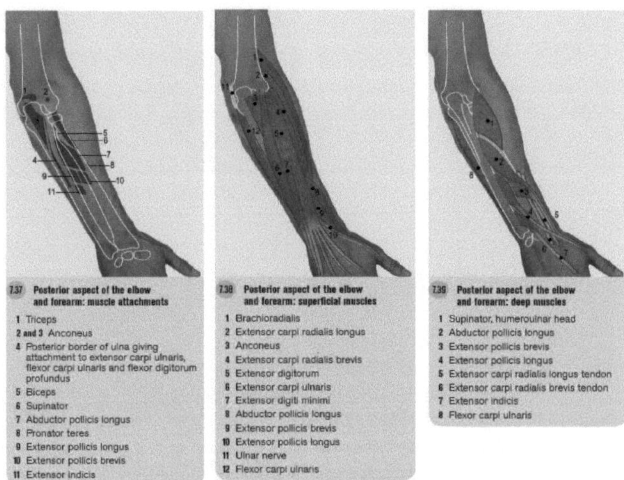

Figure 24. Superficial anatomy and surgery Behind the forearm

Tactile tendons in the back of the wrist

Abductor pollicis longus

On the outside and in front of the anatomical snuff box, it passes over the radial styloid and usually has two tendons. This tendon is associated with the Extensor pollicis brevis tendon and it is difficult to diagnose each one separately.

Extensor pollicis longus

It is located on the inside and back of the descriptive sniffer. In order to better identify the recent tendon, it is better that the thumb is in full extension, in which case the tendon can be followed to the point of adhesion to the end ligament.

Extensor carpi radialis longus

In case of resistance to wrist extension, it is immediately touched outside the Extensor pollicis longus tendon and inside the anatomical ventilator.

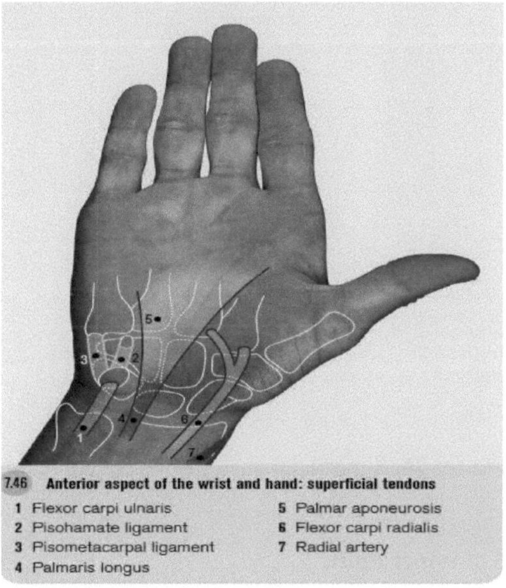

Figure 25. Superficial anatomy and surgery Wrist

Extensor carpi radialis brevis

When the thumb is loose, with resistance to wrist extension, it is immediately palpable inside the Extensor pollicis longus tendon, which attaches to the third metacarp.

Extensor digitorum, Extensor indicis and Extensor digiti minimi

The tendons of these muscles can be seen and touched on the back of the wrist and the back of the hand by opening the wrist against resistance.

Flexor carpi ulnaris

By moving towards the Pronation and moving the wrist inwards (Adduction), its tendon between the Ulnar styloid and the base of the fifth metacarp is touched. This condition is important because in conditions such as rheumatoid arthritis, when the movement to the back of the ulna increases, surgery is performed to return the tendon to its normal position.

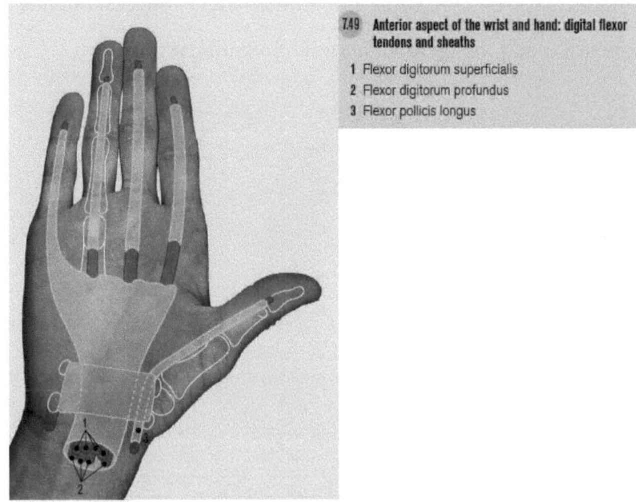

Figure 26. Superficial anatomy Wrist and palm

Cavities and spaces of upper limbs

Supraclavicular fossa

This space is located in the neck and above the middle third of the clavicle and is bounded at the front by the Sternocleidomastoid muscle (SCM) and at the back by the anterior side of the Trapezius. This space is related to the neck and will be discussed in the relevant chapter.

Infraclavicular fossa

It is located between the attachment of the pectoralis major muscle to the clavicle and the deltoid muscle, and ends in a groove called the Deltopectoral groove, which contains the cephalic vein and the deltoid artery. On the outside of this cavity and under the clavicle, the Coracoid appendage is palpable. There are also several lymph nodes (Infraclavicular nodes) inside this cavity that receive superficial lymph along the cephalic vein.

Underarm cavity (Armpit = axilla)

It is a pyramidal hole with a vertex at the top. This cavity is bounded on the outside by the arm, on the inside by the ribs and the chest wall, and on the front and back by the anterior and dorsal axillary folds. When the hand approaches the trunk with resistance (Adduction) or by pressing the hand on the hip bone, these folds become protruding and palpable.

When the upper arm is raised, the axillary region becomes a narrow groove. The anterior fold of the axilla is created by the lower side of the pectoralis major muscle, while the dorsal fold is created by the Teres major and Latissimus dorsi muscles. The inner wall of the cavity is created by the Serratus anterior and the ribs. Its outer wall consists of the upper arm bone and the Coracobrachialis muscle and the short head of the biceps.

The last two muscles in the outer wall form a distinct muscle bulge. Next to the back of this muscular ridge is the neurovascular bundle, which includes the axillary and median nerves, the ulnar, the inner lining of the forearm, and the radial of the brachial plexus. The axillary cavity is very important due to the presence of the brachial neural network, the axillary artery and vein, and the lymph nodes, each of which will be discussed in the relevant sections.

Ausculating triangle

It is the part of the chest wall that is less covered by muscles and is used to listen to lung sounds or fluid to pass through the esophagus (in cases of esophageal stricture). Theoretically, the lower side is completed by Latissimus dorsi, the outer side by the inner side of the scapula and the inner side by the lower side of the trapezius. But in practice, the phone should be placed next to the inside of the Scapula near a low angle.

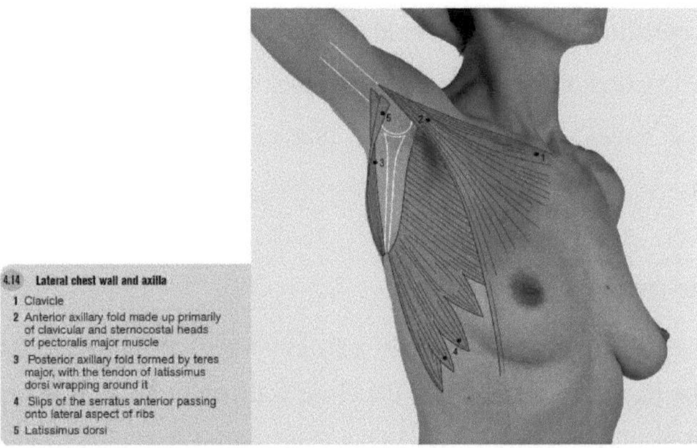

Figure 27. Superficial anatomy of the trunk muscles from the side view

Cubital fossa

Due to the presence of neurological, vascular and tendon structures at the surface and depth is of particular importance. The walls and its sides are:

A) Outside, Brachioradialis muscle.

B) Inside, the flexor muscles of the forearm, especially the pronator teres.

C) The base (upper side), the line that connects the two epicondyles of the arm.

Because both muscles attach to the radius at the bottom, the apex is at the bottom and outside. Median cubital vein (if present) passes obliquely through the surface of this cavity. This cavity is divided by the Biceps brachii tendon into two internal or external cavities or grooves:

1) **Lateral cubital groove (fossa):** Located between the Biceps tendon and the Brachioradialis muscle. The cephalic vein and the lateral cutaneous nerve of the forearm pass through the surface of this groove, and inside this cavity are the radial nerve and the radial recurrent artery.
2) **Medial cubital groove (fossa):** Located between the Pronator teres tendon and the Biceps. The basilic vein and the medial cutaneous nerve of the forearm pass

through the surface of this cavity, and inside this cavity from outside to inside are the following buildings, respectively:

A) Brachial artery

B) Median nerve

C) Ulnar recurrent arteries

The superficial and deep structures of this section are separated by Bicipital aponeurosis.

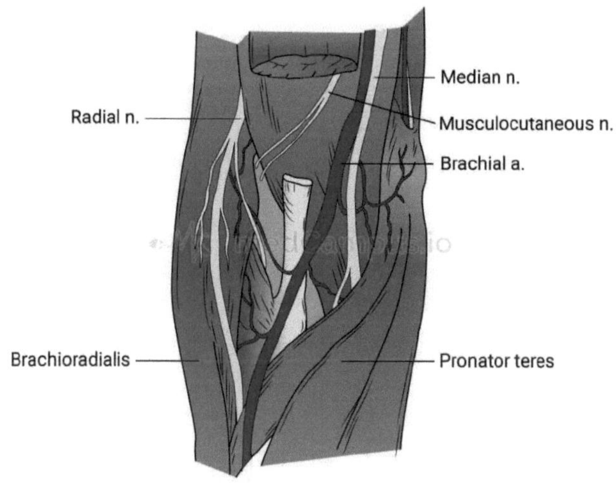

Figure 28. Arteries and veins of the elbow

Anatomical snuff box

When the thumb is fully open (Extension), this depression is visible on the outer surface of the wrist, below the lower end of the radius. This depression is bounded on the outside or front by the Extensor pollicis brevis and Abductor pollicis longus tendons and on the inside or back by the Extensor pollicis longus tendon. The Styloid protrusions of the radius, scaphoid, trapezium, and base of the first metacarp are located at the bottom of the depression, and the pulse of the radial artery can be felt deep in the depression. In addition, the superficial radial nerve and the cephalic vein cross its surface.

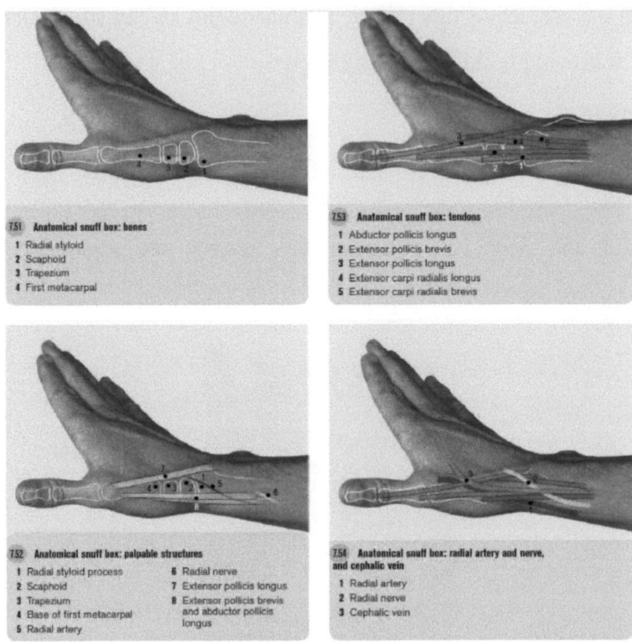

Figure 29. Lateral arteries and bones of the wrists and fingers

Wrist area

Flexor and Extensor retinaculum and transverse folds of wrist are present in this area.

A) Flexor retinaculum: A transverse band that stretches in front of the wrist and has two upper and lower sides. The surface position of the upper side can be achieved by connecting the Tubercle of scaphoid and Pisiform. This is parallel to the distal wrist crease. Tubercle of trapezium and hook of hamate must be connected to determine the position of the lower side. This side is about 4 cm lower than the upper side and can be considered parallel to the thumb that is fully open. The lower side of the retinaculum is also the surface of the deep palmar arch.

B) Extensor retinaculum: An oblique strip 2 cm wide that is located in the middle of the back of the hand. This retinaculum connects to the front of the radial styloid from the outside and to the Triquetrum and Pisiform bones from the inside.

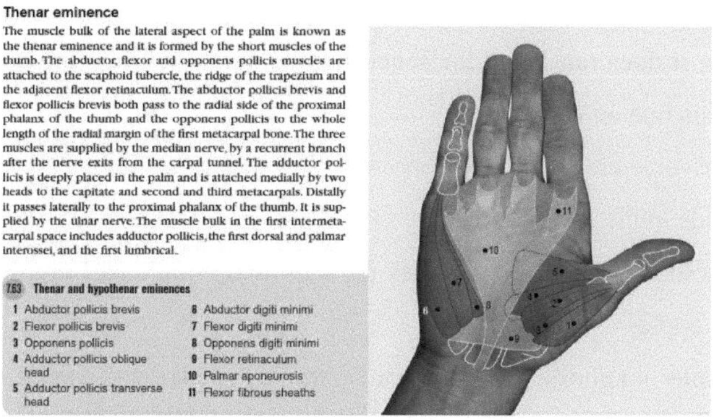

Thenar eminence

The muscle bulk of the lateral aspect of the palm is known as the thenar eminence and it is formed by the short muscles of the thumb. The abductor, flexor and opponens pollicis muscles are attached to the scaphoid tubercle, the ridge of the trapezium and the adjacent flexor retinaculum. The abductor pollicis brevis and flexor pollicis brevis both pass to the radial side of the proximal phalanx of the thumb and the opponens pollicis to the whole length of the radial margin of the first metacarpal bone. The three muscles are supplied by the median nerve, by a recurrent branch after the nerve exits from the carpal tunnel. The adductor pollicis is deeply placed in the palm and is attached medially by two heads to the capitate and second and third metacarpals. Distally it passes laterally to the proximal phalanx of the thumb. It is supplied by the ulnar nerve. The muscle bulk in the first intermetacarpal space includes adductor pollicis, the first dorsal and palmar interossei, and the first lumbrical.

7.63 Thenar and hypothenar eminences

1 Abductor pollicis brevis
2 Flexor pollicis brevis
3 Opponens pollicis
4 Adductor pollicis oblique head
5 Adductor pollicis transverse head
6 Abductor digiti minimi
7 Flexor digiti minimi
8 Opponens digiti minimi
9 Flexor retinaculum
10 Palmar aponeurosis
11 Flexor fibrous sheaths

Figure 30. Superficial anatomy of the palm

C) Wrist creases: There are three skin folds on the front surface of the wrist that are visible to most people in two folds:

1) Proximal wrist crease: At the upper limit of the synovial sheath are the flexor tendons of the fingers.

2) Middle wrist crease: Located at the level of the wrist joint.

3) Distal wrist crease: It is flush with the upper edge of the Flexor retinaculum.

Palm of the hand

There are two muscular protrusions in the palm:

A) Thenar eminence on the outside of the palm.

B) Hypothenar eminence on the inside of the palm.

The skin of the palm and the front surface of the fingers have special characteristics. For example, the skin on the palms of the hands is light and pale, even in blacks. The skin attaches tightly to the underlying fascia.

There are special folds in the palm of the hand (Flexure lines) that are better seen when bending the fingers. These folds are:

A) Radial longitudinal crease or Life line is located inside the Thenar ridge.

B) Proximal transverse crease or head line is drawn from the inside to the outside. Of course, it does not reach the inner side completely. This line connects to the previous line on the outside.

C) Distal transverse crease or heart line, which starts from the inner side of the hand and ends in the gap between the middle fingers and the index finger.

These three folds are fixed. Sometimes the following duplicates are also present in most people:

D) Intermediate longitudinal crease or Fate line is located inside the external longitudinal crease of the palm and connects to the distal transverse crease of the palm.

E) Medial longitudinal crease or fortunate line is located on the outside of the hypothenar ridge and ends at the ring finger.

The condition and interpretation of all these folds are used in the palmistary. Wrinkles on the palms of the hands in people with mental retardation, such as Mongolism syndrome, differ in composition from ordinary people. It should be added that the pattern of giving syndrome has also been found in intelligent people.

The soles of the feet and toes also have creases and ridges, and it is said that the Chinese mostly examine and examine the plantar folds.

There are also folds on the fingers that are:

A) Proximal crease: It is located about 2.5 cm below the metacarpophalangeal joint and is related to the connection of the skin to the underlying tissue.

B) Middle crease: Located on the surface of the proximal interphalangeal joint.

C) Distal crease: about 0.5 cm above the distal interphalangeal joint.

In the creases of the fingers, the skin is thinner than elsewhere, and the perforated wound is more likely to penetrate the synovial sheaths around the long flexor tendons through the crease. These creases also represent lines with minimal stretch in the skin, and therefore, these lines are ideal for surgical incisions.

There are other ridges called Papillary ridges, especially in the fingertips of the fingers, the order of these ridges, known as Dermatoglyfic, is specific to each person and is used in fingerprinting for identification.

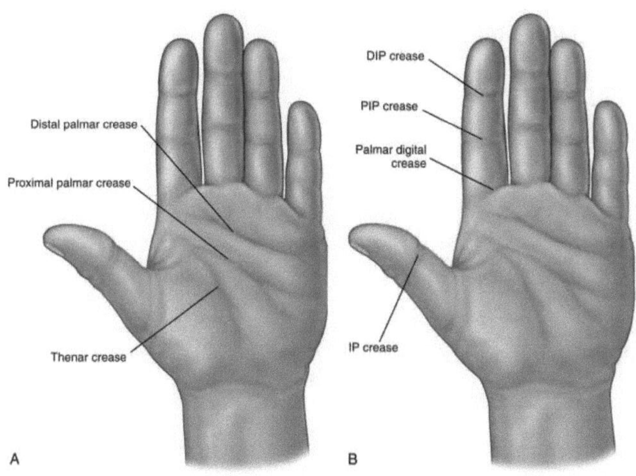

Figure 31. Superficial anatomy of the palm

Nerves of the Upper Limb

Brachial plexus

The roots (roots) and trunks (trunks) of this network are located in the back triangle of the neck and are palpable in the area that will be examined in the neck. In addition, the cords of this network can be touched in the upper part of the external Axilla wall around the Axillary artery.

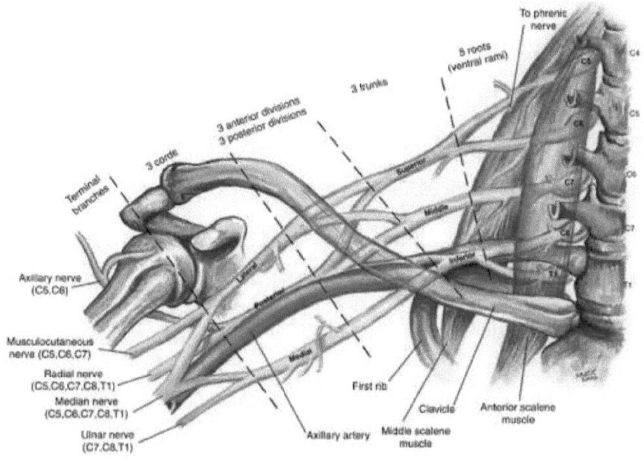

Figure 32. Brachial plexus

Armpit anesthesia locations

A) In the neck 1.5-5 cm above the pulse of the subclavian artery at the midclavicular point. In these areas, you should be careful not to pierce the lungs and sides with a needle.

B) In the outer wall of the axillary cavity behind the Coracobrachilais. In this area, you should watch out for axillary arteries.

Supraclavicular superficial nerves

These branches detach from the cervical retina (C_3-C_4), but because they attach to the skin on the shoulder, they are also discussed in the upper limbs. They are easily touched by sliding a finger on the clavicle.

How to test a nerve: Stimulate the skin on the shoulder?

Location of anesthesia: Right in the middle of the dorsal side of the Sternocleidomastoid muscle. In this area, you should watch out for the external jugular vein.

Axillary (circumflex) nerve

It detaches from the dorsal cord of the brachial plexus and innervates the deltoid and teres minor muscles and the skin above and outside the arm (on the deltoid). This nerve rotates around the surgical neck of the humerus and below the shoulder joint. The superficial position of this nerve is 4 cm below the acromial angle or 2 cm above the linear midpoint that connects the apex of the acromion to the deltoid tuberosity. This nerve may be damaged in surgical neck fractures of the humerus or dislocation of the shoulder joint.

How to test the nerve: It is better to stimulate the skin on the deltoid (upper and outer arm) because to check the deltoid operation, you should ask the patient to take his arm out (abduction), which may be unpleasant.

Nerve anesthesia site: The site of brachial plexus anesthesia.

Medial cutaneous nerve of forearm

It separates from the inner rope of the brachial plexus and descends through the groove between the biceps and triceps, and is inside the brachial artery with the ulnar nerve. This nerve, along with the basilic vein, pierces the deep fascia slightly below half the height of the arm and becomes superficial. This nerve follows the path of the said vein and may be visible in a thin person with the person's veins. Because these nerves and the external cutaneous nerve of the forearm are easily accessible, they are used for nerve grafting.

How to test a nerve: Stimulate the skin on the inside of the forearm in the middle half?

Nerve anesthesia site: In the lower third of the arm and next to the basilic vein.

Musculocutaneous nerve

It is detached from the external cord and given a nerve to the muscles of the forearm, and then pierces the deep fascia about the lower third of the arm on the outside of the arm, becomes superficial, and is known as the external cutaneous nerve of the forearm. To determine the surface direction of this nerve, connect the following points:

A) Just below and outside the Coracoid appendage.

B) Exactly outside the bicep's tendon in the Cubital cavity.

How to test the nerve: Testing the action of the forearm muscles (bending the elbow) is not very useful because despite the paralysis of the forearm muscles, the forearm muscles can still bend the forearm. So it is better to stimulate the skin of the outer half of the forearm.

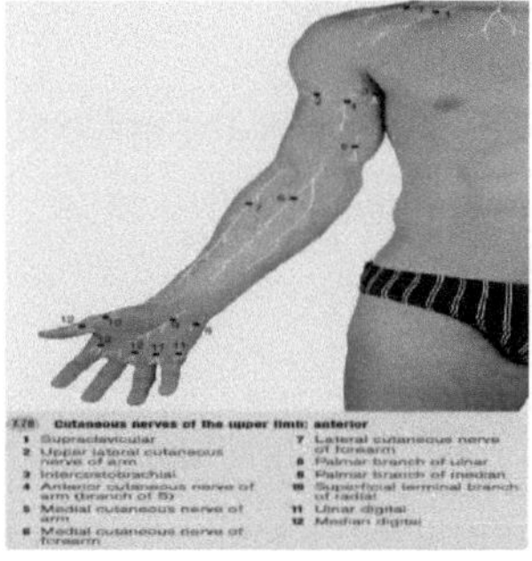

Figure 33. Superficial anatomy of the upper limb

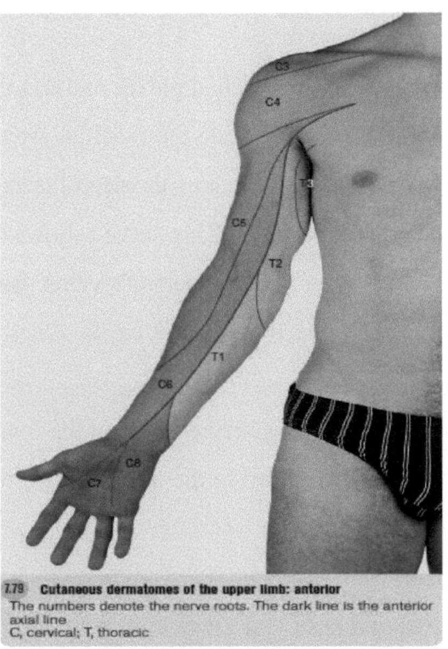

7.79 **Cutaneous dermatomes of the upper limb: anterior**
The numbers denote the nerve roots. The dark line is the anterior axial line
C, cervical; T, thoracic

Figure 34. Areas of neural distribution of the upper extremities

Lateral cutaneous nerve of forearm (external cutaneous nerve of forearm)

The extension of the nerve is musculocutaneous and is usually used for nerve grafting. This nerve is immediately outside the Biceps tendon and in the Cubital cavity. The nerve then passes through the depth of the median cubital vein near its junction to the cephalic vein and, along with the cephalic vein, innervates the radius to the styloid appendage.

How to test a nerve: Stimulate the skin on the outside of the middle half of the forearm?

Nerve anesthesia site: On the surface of the epicondyles of the arm immediately adjacent to the external Biceps tendon.

Radial nerve

The continuation of the back rope is the brachial plexus. From the medial side of the biceps muscle in front of the dorsal axilla fold, go obliquely to the back of the arm, and in the upper third that connects the deltoid site to the external epicondyle of the arm, pierce the intermuscular septum and lower the anterior condylar of the lower arm. comes. This nerve is divided into superficial and deep branches around the external epicondyle. Here we examine the nerve and its branches.

1) To determine the superficial position of the nerve in the arm, connect the following points:

A) In the medial bicipital groove behind the Coracobrachialis muscle, where the pulse of the axillary artery is felt.

B) At the junction of the middle and lower third of the line that connects the acromion appendage to the outer epicondyle of the arm.

C) One centimeter outside the biceps tendon at the level of the outer epicondyle of the arm.

It should be noted that the radial nerve can be felt at point B (about 1 to 2 cm below the deltoid site) or at the bottom of the barrow between the Triceps and Brachialis muscles. This nerve surrounds the humerus in the spiral groove and may be damaged in a fracture of the trunk of the humerus. As a result, all the extensor muscles of the wrist are paralyzed and the wrist drops. But forearm extension does not cause much damage, because the branches that come to the triceps are mainly detached before the helical groove in the axillary cavity.

How to test a nerve?

1) Irritation of the skin on the back of the arm.

2) Irritation of the skin below and outside the arm.

3) Stimulation of the skin behind the forearm in the middle half.

Location of anesthesia or electrical stimulation

1) brachial plexus anesthesia.

2) One centimeter behind and below the deltoid adhesion.

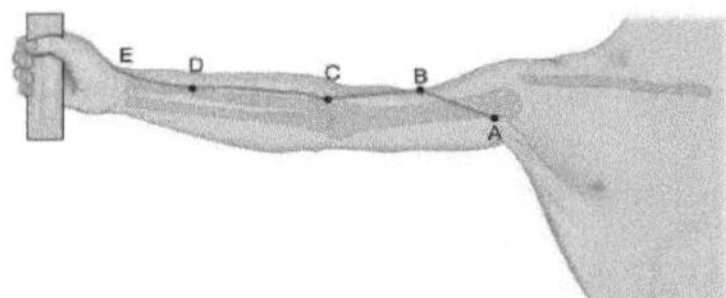

Fig. 5.9: Radial nerve.

In the forearm:

a. Mark a point medial to the brachial artery at neck of the radius (A).
b. Another point at the middle of the palmar aspect of wrist (B).
c. Join A and B.

Radial Nerve (Fig. 5.9)

In the arm:

a. A point in the lateral wall of the axilla at its lower boundary (A).
b. A point at the junction of the upper one third and lower two third of the arm along the lateral border (B).
c. A point at the level of the lateral epicondyle and lateral to the tendon of biceps (C).
d. Join points A, B and C. This is the radial nerve in the arm.

In the forearm:

d. From the point C, mark a point at the junction of the upper two thirds and the lower third of the forearm along the lateral border of the forearm (D).
e. Another point at the anatomical snuff box (E).
f. Join points C, D, and E. This is the radial nerve lying lateral to the radial artery.

Figure 35. Superficial anatomy of the radial nerve

Superficial radial nerve

It is quite sensory. To determine the position of this nerve, connect the following points:

A) One centimeter outside the biceps tendon at the level of the outer epicondyle of the arm.

B) At the junction of the lower and middle thirds of the line connecting the outer epicondyle of the arm to the styloid radius appendage.

C) In the upper part of the Anatomical snuff box.

The nerve is aneurysmally with the cephalic vein and may be damaged at the * Cutdown * of the cephalic vein.

How to test a nerve: Stimulate the skin on the first space behind the hand?

Nerve anesthesia site

1) One centimeter outside the Biceps tendon at the level of the outer epicondyle of the arm.

2) In the anatomical vein next to the cephalic vein.

Deep radial nerve

It is fully motile and, after detaching from the radial nerve, passes through the supinator and is known as the posterior interosseous. To determine the surface direction of this nerve, connect the following points:

A) One centimeter outside the biceps tendon at the level of the outer epicondyle of the arm.

B) The junction of the upper third and lower two thirds of the line connecting the radius head to the dorsal tubercle radius.

C) One centimeter below the midline of the line connecting the head of the ulna and the dorsal tubercle of the radius on the dorsal surface of the wrist.

How to test a nerve: Extension of the thumb and the rest of the fingers or wrist?

Location of electrical nerve stimulation: one centimeter outside the Biceps tendon at the level of the external epicondyle.

Posterior cutaneous nerve of forearm

It separates from the radial nerve in the spiral groove or higher. To touch this nerve, hold the radius with the index finger and the middle of the head. The little finger will mark this nerve when you move it back and forth.

How to test a nerve: Stimulate the skin behind the forearm in the middle half?

Nerve anesthesia site: 1 cm behind and below the deltoid adhesion.

Median nerve

It is separated from the external and internal ropes of the brachial plexus. To determine the surface path of this nerve, you must connect the following points:

A) Slightly below and outside the Coracoid appendage.

B) Right next to the inner end of the brachial artery in the Cubital cavity.

C) On the inside of the tendon of the Flexor carpi radialis muscle in front of the wrist.

The distance between points A and B determines the path of the nerve in the arm, the whole path of which is accompanied by the brachial artery. It is located at the top on the outside and at the bottom on the inside of the artery. In the upper half, the arm passes over the artery and is palpable. The distance between B and C shows the nerve pathway in the forearm. In the upper part, the nerve is located behind the Flexor digitorum superficialis muscle, but in the lower part of the forearm, it is located between the tendons of Palmaris longus and Flexor carpi radialis and passes behind the Flexor retinaculum and enters the palm. About 5-6 cm above the wrist, the palmar cutaneous branch separates from the palmar skin and passes through the retinaculum and goes to the palm skin. This branch is clinically important. The median nerve in the carpal tunnel syndrome is compressed and causes pain in 3.5 external fingers, but there are no neurological symptoms of the palmar cutaneous branch because it separates before the retinaculum.

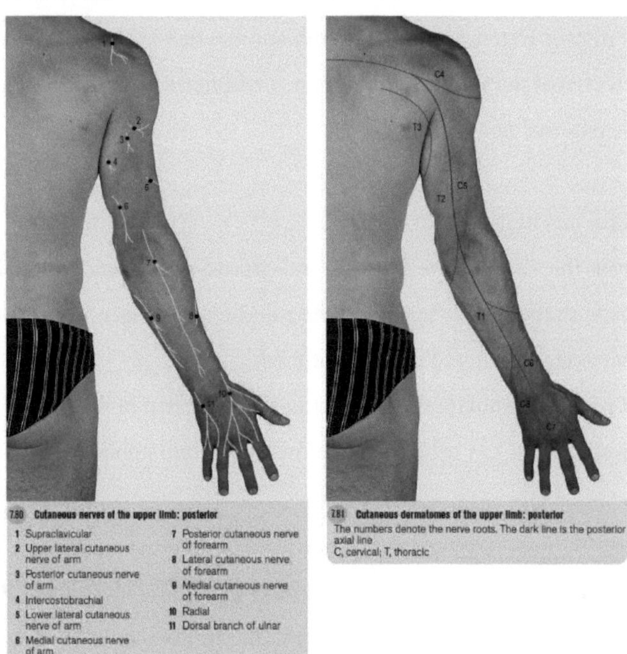

Figure 36. Superficial anatomy of the nerves behind the forearm

How to test a nerve?

1) Irritation of the skin of the thenar area of the palm.

2) Stimulation of the distal skin of the index and middle fingers.

3) Perform Thumb Opposition.

Location of anesthesia or electrical stimulation of the nerve:
1) In the elbow immediately next to the inner arm artery.
2) In the wrist between the tendons of Palmaris longus and Flexor carpi radialis.

Ulnar nerve

It originates from the inner rope, although sometimes a C_7 branch from the outer rope joins it. To determine the surface direction of the nerve, connect the following points:
A) Slightly below and outside the Coracoid appendage.
B) The middle of the inner side of the arm.
C) Behind the inner epicondyle of the arm.
D) Just outside the Pisiform bone.

It is relatively superficial in the axilla and arm between A and B and may be damaged by external injuries and compressions. It is located between the Coracobrachialis and the Triceps and then inside the Biceps along with the Brachial Artery. Go from point B to the back of the arm and behind the inner epicondyle of the arm. It is located in a tunnel created by the bones and heads of the Flexor carpi ulnaris muscle (Cubital tunnel), which may be damaged by fracture of this bone or compression by the muscle fibrosis arch (Cubital tunnel syndrome). In this place, if you put pressure on the nerve, a tingling and murmur feeling will appear on the inside of the hand. Points mark the nerve pathway in the forearm, which is located on the outside of the ulnar artery in the lower two-thirds of the forearm.

About 5-7.5 cm above the Styloid ulna of the ulna. The ulnar nerve is divided into superficial and deep branches right on the Pisiform. Ulnar nerve palsy causes both the little finger and the ring in the metacarpophalangeal joints to become hyperextension and the interphalangeal joints to flexion, resulting in a condition called the claw hand.

How to test a nerve?

1) Stimulation of the skin of the little finger for sensory fibers.

2) Hold the pencil between the fingers.

3) Due to the fact that the grip of objects in the hand (Power grip) is done obliquely and this is done by the ulnar nerve, this may be impossible in ulnar nerve damage.

4) Bring the thumb closer to all fingers (Opposition), in which case both the ulnar and median nerves are tested.

Locations of anesthesia with electrical nerve stimulation

1) Behind the inner epicondyle of the arm.

2) Immediately next to the Pisiform exterior.

Nervous skin of the upper limb

In summary, the upper extremity nerve is as follows

1. Head by Supraclavicular nerves of the cervical network.
2. The outer part of the arm at the top (on the deltoid) by the Axillary nerve and at the bottom by the Radial nerve.
3. The inner part of the forearm at the top by the medial cutaneous nerve of the arm and at the bottom by the medial cutaneous nerve of the forearm.
4. The back of the arm by the Radial nerve.
5. Outside and in front of the forearm by Lateral cutaneous nerve of forearm.
6. Inside and in front of the forearm by the medial cutaneous nerve of the forearm.
7. The back of the forearm by the posterior cutaneous nerve of the forearm.
8. Palms and fingers: 3.5 outer fingers by Median and 1.5 inner fingers by Ulnar.
9. Back of hand to Interphalangeal joint 2.5 external fingers by Superficial radial nerve and 2.5 internal fingers by Ulnar nerve. The distal band of all fingers is provided by the palm branches.

Dermatome of the upper limb

The part of the skin that is innervated by a spinal segment is called a dermatome, which is very important for testing a specific part of the spinal cord. The upper limb receives nerves from the brachial plexus (C_5-T_1). The upper limb dermatome is very simple and in the following order:

1. The outer part of the arm by the fifth piece of cervical spinal cord (C_5).
2. The outer part of the forearm and thumb by (C_6).
3. The middle finger and the middle part of the hand by (C_7) (middle branch of the brachial plexus).
4. The inside of the forearm and little finger by (C_8).
5. The inside of the arm by (T_1).

Due to the fact that the skin of the inner part of the arm is innervated by the first part of the chest (T_1) and this part also gives nerves to the heart, the heart pain shoots towards the inside of the left arm.

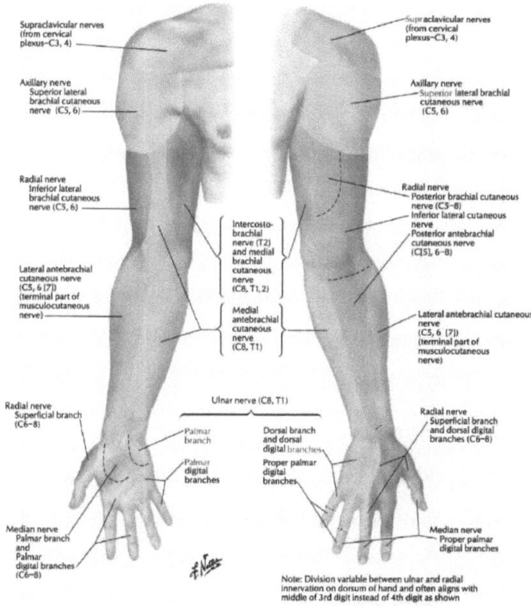

Figure 37. Anterior and posterior skin nerves of the forearm

Injection into the deltoid muscle

The axillary nerve wraps about 4 inches below the acromion around the neck of the arm surgery, but its terminal branch extends only to the outer surface of the arm. Also, the radial nerve appears between the lower third and upper two thirds between the acromion and the elbow on the outside of the arm. Therefore, it is better to inject between these two points so as not to damage the nerves.

Arteries of the Upper Limb

Axillary artery

It is a continuation of the subclavian artery. To determine its surface position, you should move your arm 90 degrees away from your torso and place your hand with your palm facing up. In this case, connect the following points to determine the path of the artery:

A) The midpoint of the lower side of the clavicle.

B) Just below the Coracoid appendage.

C) In the medial bicipital groove behind the Coracobrachialis muscle.

In this part, the pulse of the artery can be touched or the artery can be pressed on the bone to stop the blood flow during bleeding.

Brachial artery

It is a continuation of the axillary artery and descends first between the muscles of the Coracobrachialis and Triceps and then between the Triceps and Biceps and is superficial in almost all of its direction and its pulse can be felt. In the crease of the elbow, this artery passes behind the bicipital aponeurosis and divides into two terminal branches, the radial and the ulnar, in front of the neck of the radius. The following points must be connected to determine the direction of the brachial artery:

A) Medial bicipital groove behind the Coracobrachialis muscle.

B) One centimeter below the midline of the line that connects the two epicondyles of the arm in front of the elbow. This point is located right next to the inside of the Biceps tendon. Here, the pulse of the artery is easily felt and is usually where the phone is placed to take blood pressure.

When taking blood from this artery in the elbow cavity, care must be taken not to damage the median nerve, which is located immediately next to the inside of the artery.

Radial artery

The continuation is the brachial artery. In the lower third, the forearm is superficial and is placed between the Brachioradialis and Flexor carpi radialis tendons in the pulse groove, then enters the anatomical ventricle from the depth of the Abductor pollicis longus tendon. Finally, after passing through the depth of the Extensor pollicis longus tendon and from the first space between the metacarpals, it enters the palm of the hand and participates in the formation of the arterial arch of the deep palm. The pulse of the artery can also be felt in the anatomical area of the anus. To determine the surface direction of this artery, the following points must be connected:

A) One centimeter below the midpoint of the line where he connects the epicondyle of the arm in front of the elbow.

B) In front of the lower end of the radius between the Brachioradialis and Flexor carpi radialis tendons.

C) In the middle of the descriptive sniffer.

D) At the upper end of the first space between the metacarpals.

Ulnar artery

The larger branch is the brachial artery, which is deeper in its path. To determine the surface direction of this artery, connect the following points:

A) One centimeter below the midline of the line that connects the two epicondyles of the arm in front of the elbow (the end of the brachial artery).

B) The junction of the upper and middle third of the line that extends from the inner epicondyle of the arm to the pisiform bone.

C) Just outside Pisiform.

The pulse of the artery is palpable outside the Flexor carpi ulnaris tendon, and the ulnar nerve is located immediately next to the inside of the artery.

Superficial palmar arch

It consists of the ulnar artery and the superficial branch of the radial artery. To determine the surface direction of this arc, connect the following points:

A) Just outside the Pisiform bone.

B) Hook of hamate.

C) Proximal palmar crease.

D) In the middle of the Thenar ridge.

The distal end of this arch touches the upper crease of the palm.

Deep palmar arch

It consists of the radial artery and the deep branch of the ulnar artery. To determine the surface direction of this arc, connect the following points:

A) Just below the Hook of hamate.

B) The distal end of the Flexor retinaculum.

C) Four centimeters on the outside of point A.

This arch is about one centimeter higher than the arch of the superficial palm and is located at the lower level of the thumb that is fully open.

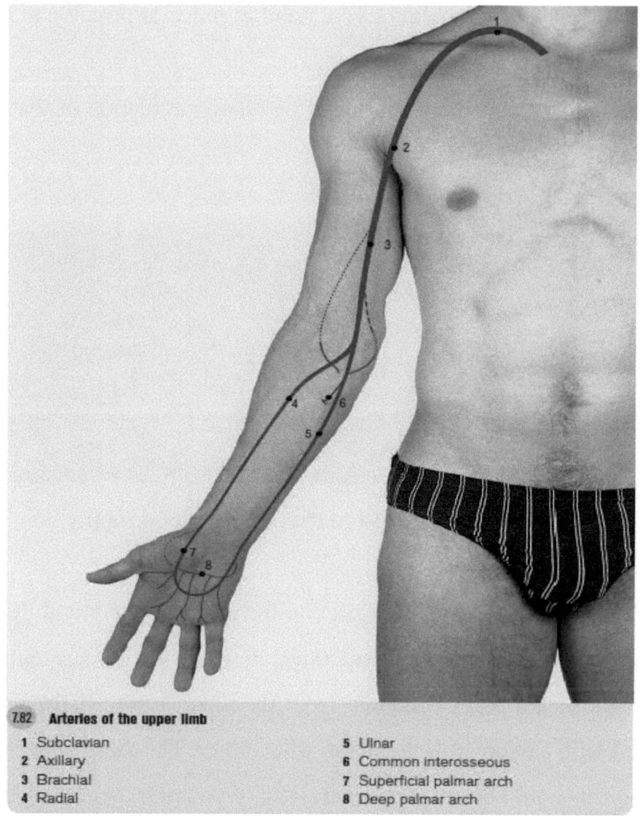

Figure 38. Surgical and superficial anatomy of the forearm and palm arteries

Note: Although it is commonly considered in the anatomy of the palmar arch between the radial and ulnar arteries. But it is clinically important that this arc is present in only 36% of people. The ulnar artery is also the main artery that nourishes the superficial tissues of the palm in most cases. Sometimes the main artery of the superficial tissues of the palm is radial. Allen's test is used to determine which artery is the main source of nutrition.

Allen's test

To determine the relative size of the main artery of the palm, the following steps should be performed:

A) Press your fingers into the palm of your hand as much as possible to get the blood out of the superficial tissue of the palm.
B) Press the radial artery in the wrist to cut the blood circulation of that artery to the palm of the hand.

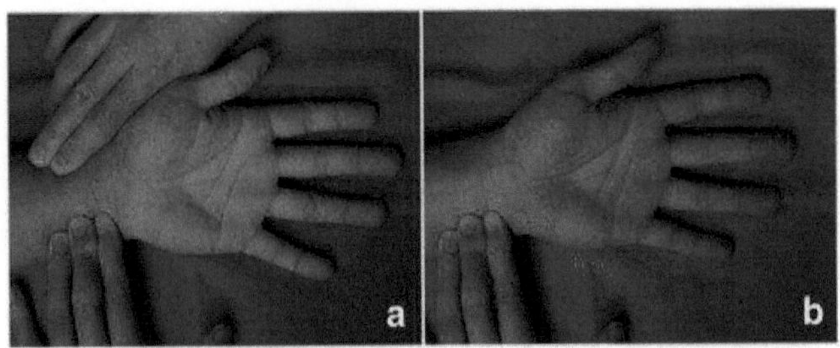

Figure 39. Allen test to check hand blood supply

C) Open your fingers as you apply pressure to the artery. If the blood flow is fast and the palm quickly becomes bloody and thick, it is clear that the nutrition of the superficial tissue of the palm is mainly from the ulnar artery. If the palm becomes bloody and red with a delay, it is the main radial artery. The same test can be done for the ulnar artery. It should be noted that normally, if you press your finger on the palm of your hand and then open your fingers, the palm will immediately become bloody and full of color. This test is used during hemodialysis (Haemodialis).
This test should be performed if they want to insert a needle that carries blood from the body into the device into the radial artery. If the superficial tissue of the palm takes blood mainly from the radial and a needle is inserted into the radial artery, the palm becomes anemic. In this case, the needle must be inserted after the superficial branch of the palm separates from the radial artery (for example, in the Anatomical snuff box).

Veins of the Upper Limb

There are two categories of deep and superficial veins. Deep veins are usually paired and there are two deep veins for each artery. The superficial path of the deep veins is

similar to that of the arteries. The superficial veins mainly consist of the posterior vein network and the two Cephalic and Basilic veins.
In lean individuals, superficial veins bulge and become visible when the upper limb is suspended. However, in obese people and those whose veins are not clear for any reason, it is possible to make the veins more distinct and prominent by tying a blood pressure monitor arm around the arm or holding the arm by hand. It should be noted that superficial veins have a lot of variation in people and even in the two hands of one person there are obvious differences.

Dorsal venous network or arch behind the hand

There is a venous network behind each finger that forms the dorsal digital veins. These veins then join together to form the Metacarpal veins, of which there is one in each space. Eventually, these veins together form the network or arch of the posterior hand. A vein separates from each side of the network, called the cephalic vein on the outside and the basilic vein on the inside.

Basil vein

It starts from the inside of the venous arch behind the hand. Walk slightly behind the forearm and then forward and up inside the forearm to reach the medial cubital groove. Here it travels along the medial cutaneous nerve of the forearm and, just below half the height of the arm with the nerve, pierces the deep fascia and deepens and extends as the axillary vein. In the Cubital cavity, it is connected to the Cephalic vein by a vein called the median cubital.

Cephalic vein

It starts from the outside of the venous arch behind the hand. It then passes over the Anatomical snuff box and ascends from the outside of the forearm. In the Cubital area, it is connected to the Basilic vein by the median cubital vein. The cephalic vein continues to ascend in the lateral bicipital groove in the arm and enters the deltopectoral groove, at the end of which the perforated clavicle fascia is drained and drained into the axillary vein. In the anatomy it is accompanied by the superficial radial nerve and in the lateral cubital groove it is associated with the lateral cutaneous nerve of the forearm.

Median cubital vein

In some people, it is present in the anterior region of the elbow instead of the cephalic and basilic veins.

Median vein of forearm

In some people, instead of the median cubital vein in front of the forearm, there is this vein between the two cephalic and basilic veins, which eventually connects to the cephalic vein by a branch called the median cephilic and to the basilic by another branch called the median basilic.

These two connecting veins, the Cephalic and Basilic veins, together form an M-shaped state known as the venous M.

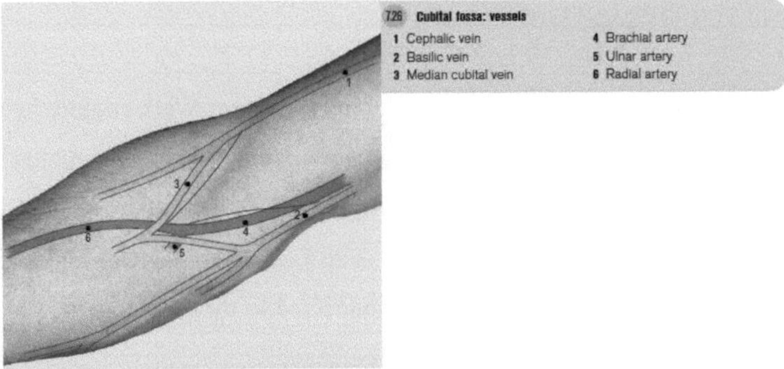

Figure 40. Elbow vessels

Venous valves

If you place your finger on a superficial vein and gently pull it down, there will be a significant bulge in the vein wherever there is a valve.

Clinical tip

The superficial veins of the upper extremities are frequently used for intravenous injections, venous blood sampling, and cut-down. Median cubital or M veins are usually the most accessible veins. Due to the path of these veins and close proximity to the median nerve and brachial artery and other reasons, it is better to use the back of the hand and Cephalic and Basilic veins in the lower forearm during injections.

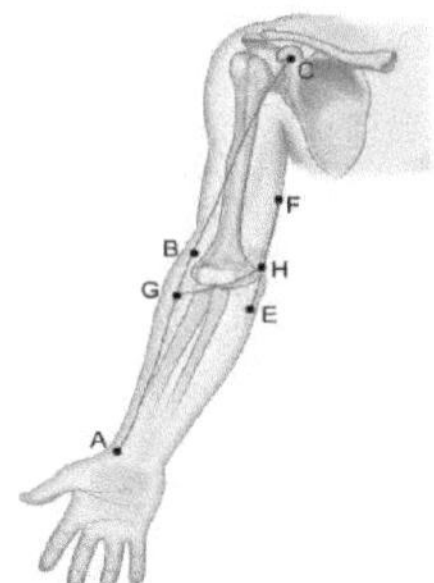

Fig. 5.13: Cephalic, basilic and median cubital vein. (ABC: Cephalic vein; EF: Basilic vein; GH: Median cubital vein).

Figure 41. Superficial anatomy of the veins of the upper extremities

Chapter III

Superficial Anatomy of the Lower Limb

Bone signs of the lower limb

Hip bone symptoms

Iliac crest: It is the interface between the waist and the hips, its entire length can be felt in the lower margin of the waist. It leads from the front to the anterior superior iliac spine (ASIS) and from the back to the posterior superior iliac spine (PSIS). This ridge is harder and more uneven in men and has more inward curvature at the front end, but in women it is more vertical.

Upper anterior iliac spine (ASIS): The anterior end of the iliac crest is easily palpable in the 12 cm area of the midline of the body. In addition, ASIS is the level of PSIS, the sacral vertebra (S_2), the sacroiliac joint, and the lowest level of the subarachnoid space.

Tubercle of Iliac crest: The short bulge touches the outer surface of the iliac crest, 5 cm behind the ASIS. This bulge is flush with the fifth lumbar vertebra (L_5).

Highest point of iliac crest: It is located slightly behind the midline of the Iliac crest and is located at the level of the space between the thorny edges of the third and fourth lumbar vertebrae (L_3-L_4). Used as a marker for locating cerebrospinal fluid (Lumbar puncture).

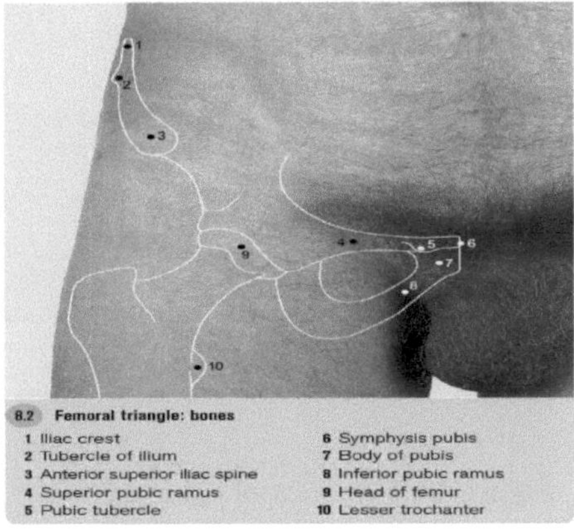

Figure 42. Femoral triangle

Upper iliac hedgehog (PSIS)

It is not easy to touch, but its position can be determined in 4 cm of the midline below the skin dimple in the lower back and upper part of the buttocks, which is level with the second sacral vertebra (S_2) and ASIS. The skin indentation is a good sign for drawing a bone marrow puncture sample from the ilium, which should be inserted into the ilium about one centimeter lower than this indentation.

Symphysis pubis

At the lower end of the abdomen is located in the middle line (along the navel). The fingers may be able to touch the oblique margin and the body of the pubis bone. The upper bouts featured two cutaways, for easier access to the higher frets, and the lower bouts featured two cutaways, for easier access to the higher frets.

Pubic crest

The rounded and upper side of the trunk is the pubis bone, which extends 2.5 cm outwards from the symphysis pubis. It crosses the spermatic cord in men and the round ligament in women. If you place your fingers on the upper margin of the Symphysis Pubic and pull it outwards, this ridge will be touched.

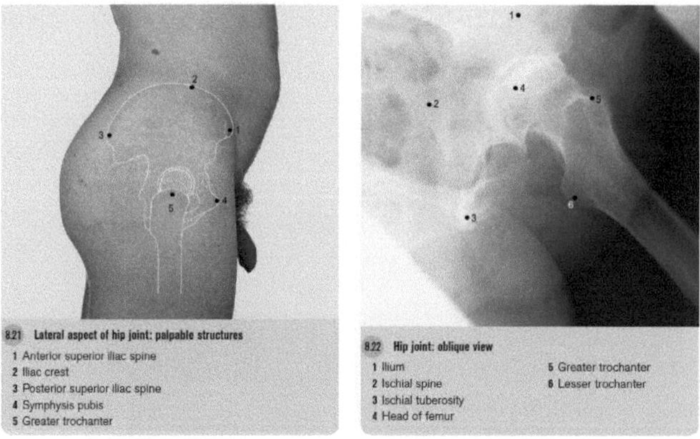

Figure 43. Side view of hip and pelvis

Pubic tubercle

It is a thick bulge that touches the outer end of the pubic crest and is 2.5 cm away from the top of the pubic symphysis. This bulge is easily felt in the skin of the scrotum in men and can be felt in women through the outer side of the labia major. This protrusion can also be felt by moving the finger above the adductor longus muscle tendon.

Ischial tuberosity

In the standing position (thigh extension) it is covered by the Gluteus maximus muscle, but when the hip joint is bent (for example, in the sitting position), this protrusion protrudes from under the lower lip of the said muscle and becomes palpable. This protrusion is located 5 cm from the midline and 5 cm above the gluteal fold.

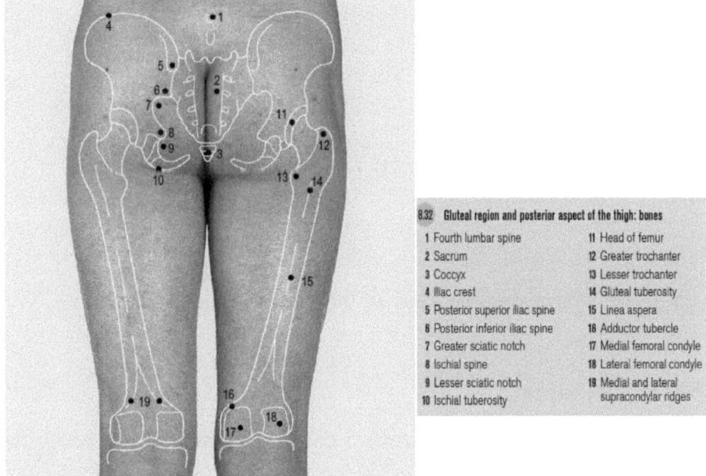

Figure 44. Superficial anatomy of the bones behind the pelvis and thigh

Thigh bone signs (Femur)

Head of femur

If you attach (ASIS) to the Symphysis pubis and consider its midpoint, then place your finger at a distance about the width of a thumb below that point and press firmly, rotating the lower limb of the femur head downward. The finger is touched.

Greater trochanter

The bulge on the outside of the upper thigh, which is easily felt in the front of the gluteal cavity, especially in thin people. The depression is located below the middle of the Iliac Crest. These bulges form the widest part of the pelvic region in thin men. In women, due to the presence of fat, the widest part of the area is slightly lower. This is also true for muscular men due to muscle mass.

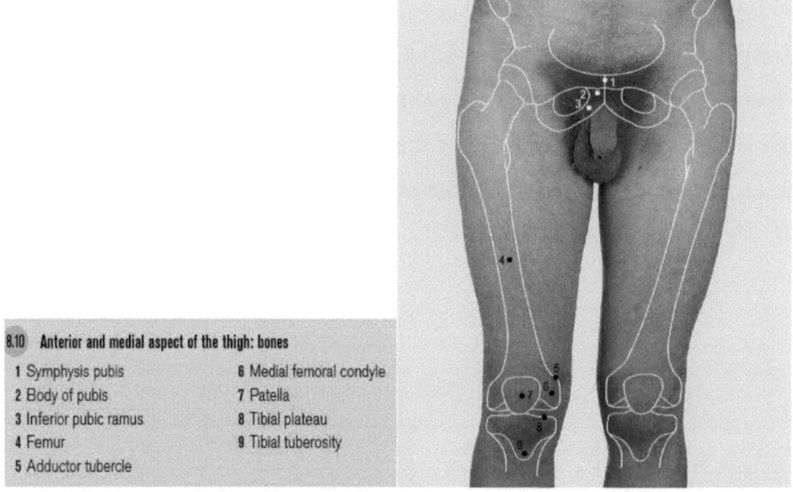

Figure 45. Superficial and anterior view of the bones of the lower limb

Ways to touch Greater trochanter

A) From the Tubercle of Iliac creste: come down 5 cm (4 fingers wide) to reach the ridge of the bone.

B) Place the thumb on the highest part of the Iliac Crest, draw a circle, marking the passage of the middle finger of the Greater trochanter.

C) Connect ASIS to Ischial Tuberosity. The intersection of the lower third and upper two thirds of the line will determine the Greater trochanter.

D) About 12 cm below the highest part of the Iliac Crest.

It should be noted that this protrusion is better felt when abduction of the hip joint. It can be uncomfortable when the person is lying on their side on the bed surface. The upper limit of the Greater trochanter is level with the center of the femoral head, the upper limit of the pubis and the apex of the sacrum in the male, or the apex of the coccyx in the female, which is above them in the abduction position.

Important lines around the pelvis

Chien's Lines

If you connect the highest point of the iliac crest, the tubercle of the iliac crest, the ASIS, and the greater trochanter of one side of the body to the eponymous points of the opposite side, lines that all must be parallel to each other are called Chien's Line.

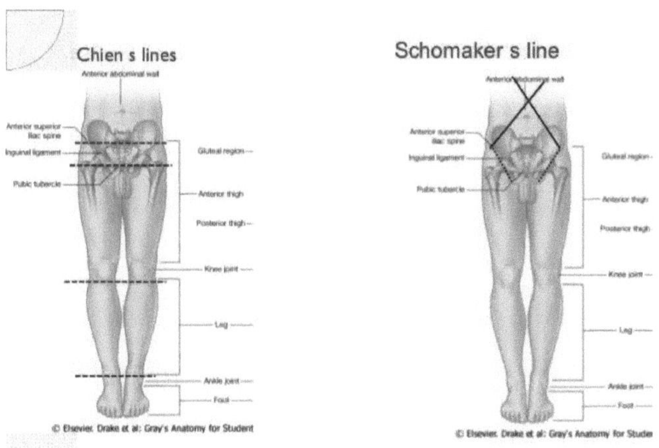

Figure 46. Pelvic surface lines

In a short time, one of the limbs may not be parallel to each other. If the lines between ASIS and the Greater trochanter are parallel, the problem is with the lower level of the Greater trochanterc. If the distance between the ASIS and the medial malleolus is not equal. One of the limbs is shorter. To determine the exact location of the short, it should be measured in the area between the Greater trochanter and the ASIS, then the ASIS to the tibial tuberosity (Tibia edge or inner side of the patella) and from here to the tip of the inner ankle.

Nelaton's line

In the anatomical position, draw a line that reaches ASIS to Ischial tuberosity by rotating the hip circumference. This line runs through the middle of the upper margin of the Greater trochanter and the center of the Acetabulum cavity and is of medical importance.

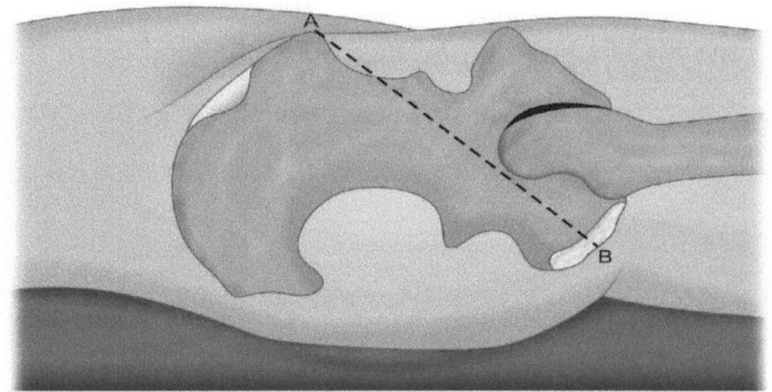

Nelaton's line. (A: Anterior superior iliac spine; B: Ischial tuberosity).

Figure 47. Nelatons line

Schomaker's line

Is a line drawn from the Greater trochanter to ASIS? If you continue this line on both sides of the top, they will intersect at the top of the umbilicus.

Bryent's triangle

If the person on the bed is supine, first connect the ASIS to the Greater trochanter. Then draw a vertical line from top to bottom from ASIS, and finally connect the Greater trochanter to the vertical line with a horizontal line. In lesions such as hip dislocation, this triangle is distorted compared to the opposite triangle, resulting in a reduced triangle depression.

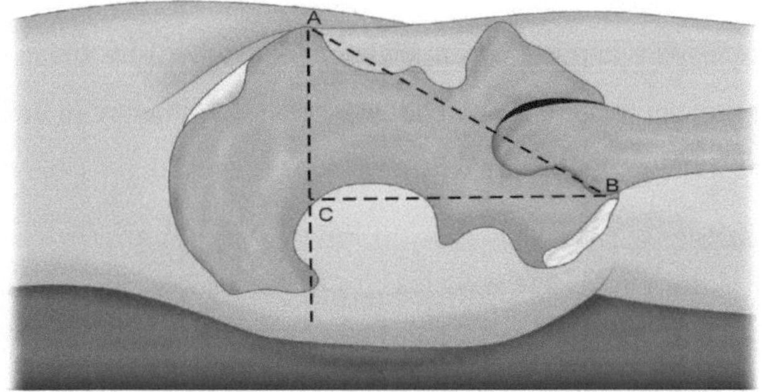

Bryant's trianle. (A: Anterior superior iliac spine; B: Greater trochanter).

Figure 48. Bryants triangle

Lesser trochanter

The Greater trochanter is not easily touched, but when lying on the prone position, it is difficult to touch with intense deep pressure on the middle of the gluteal fold in the inward rotation position and thigh extension.

Condyles of femur

When the knee is bent, the upper edge of these condyles may be felt as a prominent ridge on either side of the patella. Especially the external condyle is palpable on the outside of the Patella and in its depth. In the center of each condyle is a bulge that corresponds to the epicondyle.

Adductor tubercle

Move the thigh away from the midline of the body and rotate it outwards, then bend the knee 90 degrees (place one leg on the thigh or on the other knee). In this case, the protrusion can be felt at the bottom of the inner condyle of the thigh. The adductor magnus muscle tendon may be traced to the bulge.

Patella bone signs

When the knee is straight and the quadriceps femoris muscle is relaxed, the patella can be easily seen and touched in front of the knee or the lower side, and in front of the knee it can be moved from side to side and slightly up and down. Moved. The patella in the knee extension is about 2-2.5 cm with the tibial tuberosity and in the knee flexion is about 5 cm. In lean people, the patella is the clearest structure in the knee and is flat in the form of a bulge. In people with muscular bodies, the Vastus medialis muscle covers the upper part of the inner edge of the patella, but the lower part of the inner edge and the entire outer edge are clear. In obese people, the patella disappears in superficial fat but is still palpable subcutaneously in the center. The bony protrusions on the outside of the patella and the stretching of the Vastus medialis prevent it from dislocating outwards. The quadriceps tendon above the patella and the patellar ligament below are palpable.

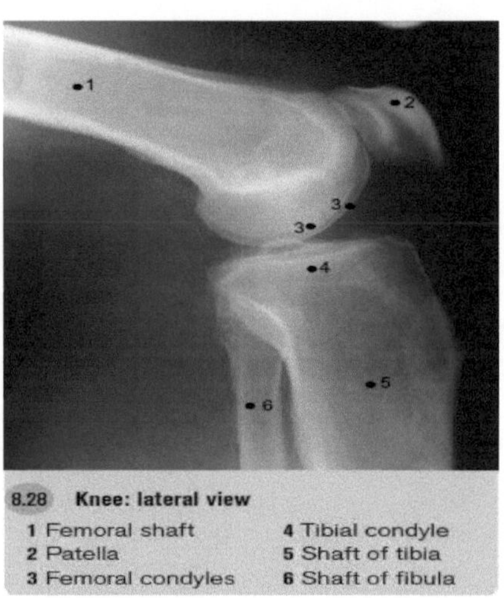

Figure 49. Knee: Lateral niew

Symptoms of tibia

Tibial tuberosity

It is located at the upper end of the anterior margin of the Tibia, 5 cm from the bent knee of the patella and 2-2.5 cm from the right knee. At the bottom is the quadriceps tendon, and at the top is a bursa between the tendon and the bone. Between this bony protrusion and the skin is a bursa called the Superficial Infra Patellar, which, if inflamed, can lead to a condition called Clergyman's Knee or Housemaid's knee, which can lead to excessive kneeling. When kneeling, this bony protrusion is placed on the ground. Above the tibial tuberosity and toward the patellar ligament, there is a dimple in which the articular space can be touched above the sharp edge of the tibial condyle.

Condyles of tibia

The front and sides of the patellar ligament are touched, especially when the knee joint is bent. In knee resistance flexion, the anterior edge of these condyles is palpable in the cavity in which the patellar ligament is located. The internal condyle is palpable below the knee joint.

Anterior side of Tibia

The front side is sharp and can be easily touched under the skin from Tibinl tuberosity to the front of the inner ankle.

Internal surface of Tibia

It is completely subcutaneous and is felt from the surface of the tibial tuberosity to the inner ankle.

Medial malleolus

If you continue down the inner surface of the Tibia, you will see this distinct and palpable bulge that is larger, forward and higher than the outer ankle. But the bottom end is not sharp.

Symptoms of fibula

Head

It is 2-3 cm below the surface of the knee joint and at the same level as the upper part of the tibial tuberosity and can be easily touched on the outer back of the knee. If you follow the biceps femoris tendon downwards, you will reach the head of this bone.

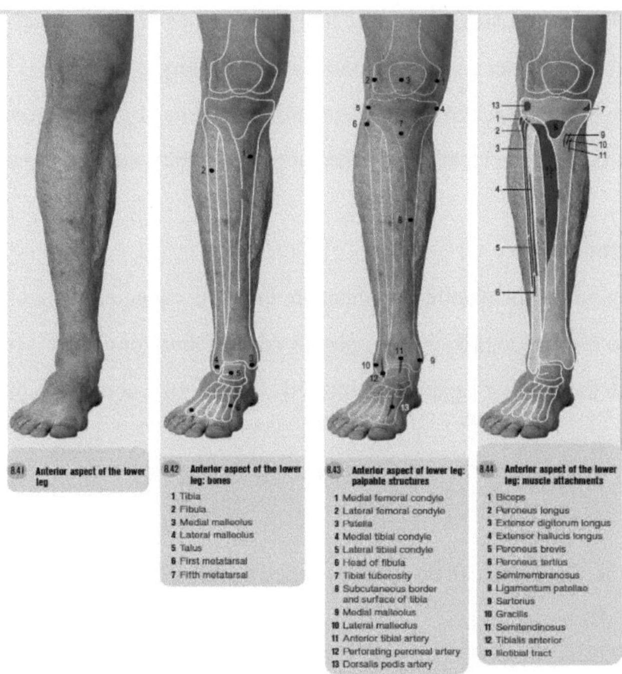

Figure 50. Superficial anatomy of the anterior leg bones

Neck of the fibula

It is touched below the head and by sliding a finger around it, the common peroneal nerve may be touched.

Body of Fibula

Only the distal part is subcutaneous and palpable and the rest is covered by muscles.

Lateral malleolus

It is clearly visible on the outer surface of the foot and is located behind and below the inner ankle. Its tip is sharp and is about 1.25 cm (half an inch) lower than the inner ankle.

Palpable bony protrusions of the ankle and foot

Peroneal tubercle

It is felt on the outer surface of the calcaneus and about 2.5 cm below and slightly in front of the external ankle. By turning the foot inward (Inversion), the tendons of Peroneus longus and brevis can be touched at the top and bottom of this ridge.

Talus (frame)

The front of the external ankle may be touched just before the neck, but if the foot is turned inwards (inversion), the talus head can be felt as a prominent protrusion on the upper and outer surface of the foot and about 3-4 cm in front of the external ankle. But in the midposition position, it is covered by the extensor digitorum brevis muscle. On the inside of the foot, the head of the talus occupies the space between the Sustentaculum tali and the Tuberosity of the navicular, and even if the foot is in Eversion, it touches under the inner ankle. If you draw a line between the inner ankle and the Tuberosity of the navicular, the head of the talus is in the middle of this line. In cases where the patient's foot is flat (flat foot), the head of the talus bone is prominent on the inside.

Sustentaculum tali

About 2.5 cm below the tip of the inner ankle may be touched. This bulge may not be felt in everyone, but it is important in terms of anatomy and is where the Spring ligament connects. Problems in this area can lead to flat feet to some extent.

Heel bone (Calcaneus)

In thin people, the lower end of the heel bone can be felt on the outside. The lower surface is covered by Plantar aponeurosis and the soleus muscles and is not easily touched.

Tuberosity of navicular

This bulge can be felt about 2.5 cm in front of the inner ankle in the middle of the way between the back of the heel and the root of the big toe (thumb). This bulge is located about 2.5 cm in front of the Sustentaculum tali. The Tibialis posterior tendon that attaches to it may also be palpable by turning the foot inward.

Cuboid (cube)

It is difficult to touch and may be indistinctly palpable behind the base of the fifth metatarsus.

Medial cunieform (inner nail)

It is vaguely felt between the Tuberosity of the navicular and the base of the first metatarsus.

Rule of the first metatarsus

It can be touched on the back of the foot. This bulge creates a large knob (Large knob) in some people, which sometimes causes compression and discomfort in the shoe.

Head of the first metatarsus

It causes a bulge on the inside of the foot, which is called the Ball of foot, and it is completely felt when the foot is straight (Extension) and especially when the thumb angle is increased (Hallux valgus). When the big toe is moved by the hand, the sesamoid bones may be touched beneath it.

Base of 5th metatars

It has a tubercle that may be felt in the middle of the outer side of the foot, and in some people their shoes may also protrude.

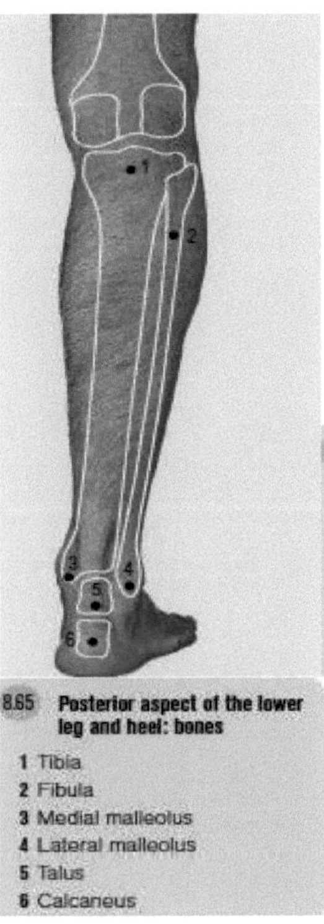

Figure 51. Superficial anatomy of the bones behind the leg

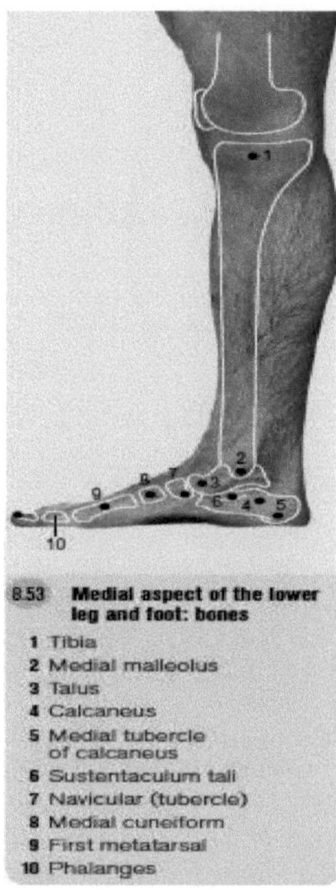

Figure 52. Superficial anatomy of the inner facade of the leg

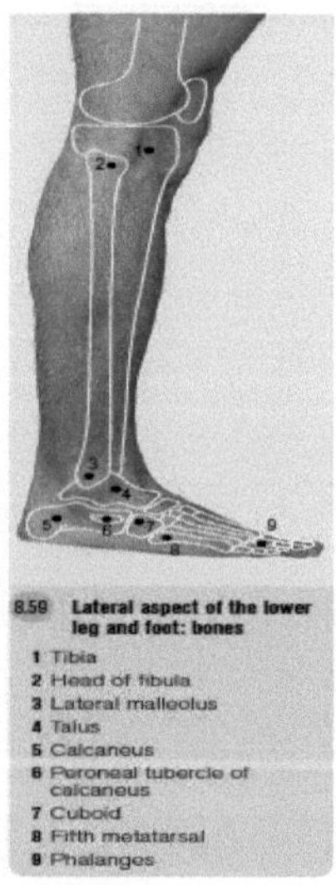

Figure 53. Superficial anatomy of the exterior of the leg

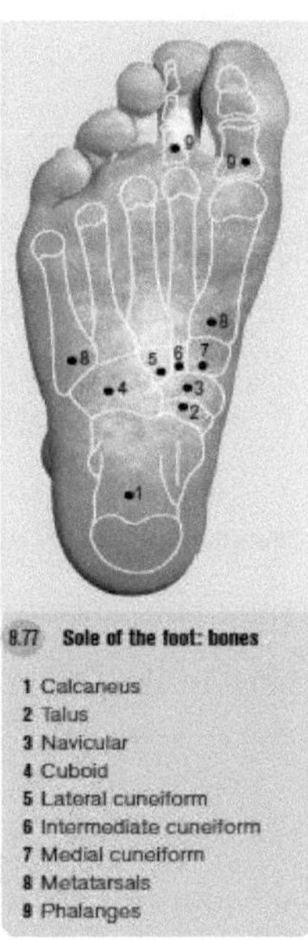

Figure 54. Superficial anatomy of the sole of the foot

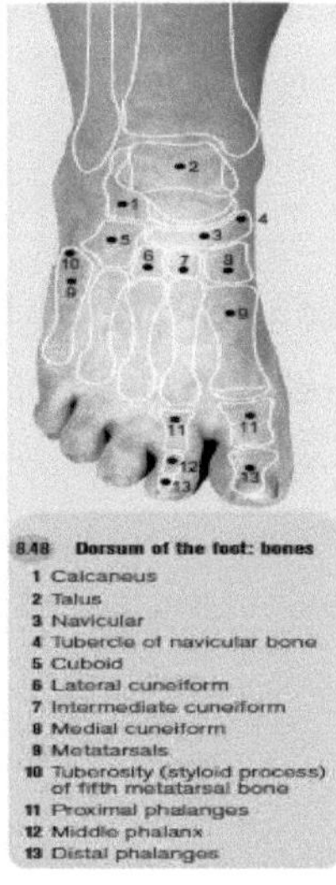

Figure 55. Superficial anatomy of the anterior view of the ankle

Joints of the lower limb

Hip joint

From the midpoint between the ASIS and the Symphysis pubis, pull 2.5-5.5 cm down and out, the center of the hip is obtained or about 1.2 cm below the midpoint of the inguinal ligament.

Knee joint

It can be felt in the narrow space between the thigh and tibia and in the indentations on the inside and outside of the patella. This surface is about 3 cm above the tibial tuberosity and 2.5-3 cm above the head of the fibula.

Tibial collateral ligament

It can be touched right inside the knee joint. Laxity This ligament is very common and may rupture in injuries (such as football). For the examination, hold the foot directly in the hand and ask the person to relax the muscles that control the knee. This ligament is tested by pressing on the outside of the knee. Some people may have joint laxity, in which case it is necessary to compare both legs.

Fibular collateral ligament

This ligament is smaller and harder to touch. Place the ankle on the opposite knee to touch it. In this case, the iliotibial tract relaxes and the ligament is easier to touch.

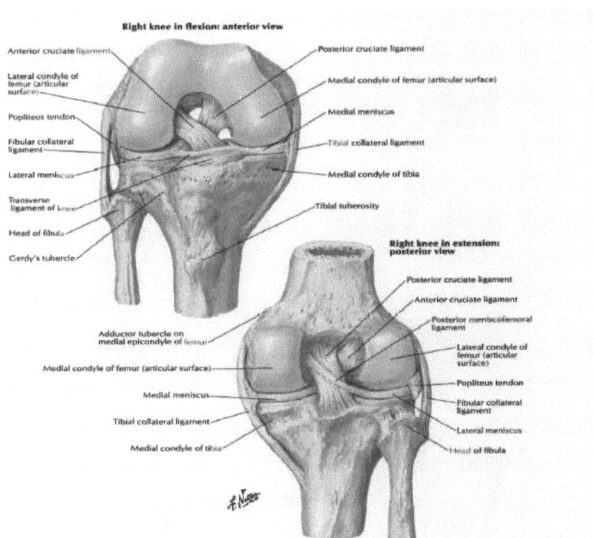

Figure 56. Menisci and knee ligaments

Meniscus

The internal meniscus is touched on the anterior side of the tibial collateral ligament. In order to touch it better, you have to passively turn the Tibia bone inwards. When the inner meniscus ruptures, the area inside the joint is painful to the touch. It is more difficult to touch the external meniscus, but it may be felt when the patient's knee is bent. Menisci are generally felt between the patellar ligament and the collateral ligament.

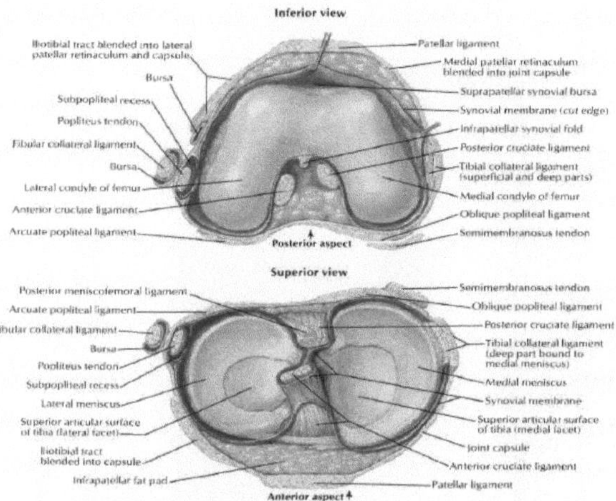

Figure 57. Menisci and knee ligaments

Cruciate ligaments

These ligaments provide internal stability to the knee area and prevent the femur from sliding forward on the tibia, and especially when descending a mountain or hill, they do not allow the femur to be in front of the tibia. These ligaments tighten completely in the position of full knee flexion and extension, and in the midflexion position of the knee, they are loose and can twist sharply. To test the cruciate ligaments, bend the knee about 90 degrees and fix the sole of the foot on the ground. Then grab the top of the leg and push it back and forth. If the ligaments are healthy, the knee should not move more than a few millimeters.

Knee angulation

In women, the pelvis is wider than in men. As a result, the heads of the femurs move further apart but at the knees so that the lower legs (legs) are vertical and parallel. Therefore, there is a small vertical angle between the thigh and the tibia, which is more common in women. If the ligaments and muscles are weak, especially due to an internal injury or due to overweight, this angle will increase and create a condition called Genu valgus. Therefore, when the knees are in contact. In women, the legs are spaced apart, and if you try to keep your feet in contact with each other, your knees will be compressed or even overlapped.

Injection into the knee joint

To inject the drug into the knee joint, the drug must be injected outside the quadriceps tendon and above the patella into the suprapatellar bursa.

Ankle joint: First, touch the two inner and outer ankles and come up 1.5 cm to the inside of the inner ankle and 2.5 cm to the top of the outer ankle. Then draw a line from these two points. This line marks the articular surface of the ankle.

The ligaments of this joint are:

1) Anterior fibular ligament: With inversion and plantar flexion, the foot may be palpable. This ligament is usually caught and sensitive in the inversion sprain of the foot.

2) Posterior talofibular ligament: Attaches to the Sustentaculum tali from the apex of the inner ankle. By turning the foot inwards, this ligament becomes elongated and palpable.

3) Calcaneo fibular ligament (Deltoid): not touched but caught in sprains.

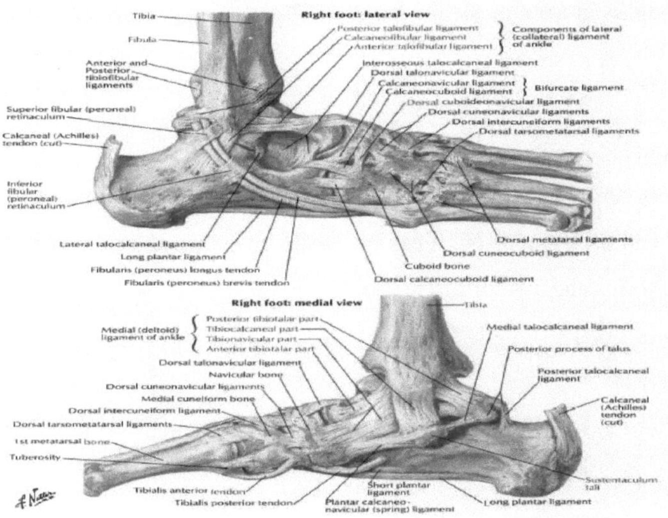

Figure 58. Floor and ankle ligaments

Muscles of the lower limb

Muscles of the front of the thigh

Tailoring (Sartorius)

By bending the thigh, turning the thigh outward and bending the knee, it is determined to put one foot on the other to do this.

Tensor fascia lata

If the patient is lying on his side and his knee is straight, it is characterized by resistance to flexion and abduction of the hip joint. This muscle and Sartorius are placed together in the shape of the number 8, the apex of which is ASIS.

Iliotibial tract

It is located on the outside of the thigh. This strip is almost visible at the lower junction with the Tibia. The dorsal side of this band should not be confused with the Biceps femoris muscle tendon, because the biceps tendon is located a short distance behind it.

Quadriceps femoris

It is a large mass in front of the thigh and has 4 heads, only three of which can be felt and seen:

Rectus femoris

If the thigh is bent 90 degrees and the knee is bent 30 degrees, if resistance is given to hip flexion and knee extension, it can be felt in the 8-shaped space created by the two muscles Sartorius and Tensor fascia lata.

Vastus lateralis

Rectus femora's is touched on the outside with resistance to straightening the knee (Extension).

Vastus medialis

With resistance of the knee extension, its muscle mass is easily seen on the inside of the Patella. This part gets nervous because of the extensor and the maintenance of the knee joint separately. If this muscle is paralyzed, because it is responsible for stabilizing the knee joint, it leads to synovitis of the knee, thus reducing protection even in light exercise such as walking. This muscle is the first part of the quadriceps muscle that suffers from atrophy after paralysis and is the last part that returns to its original state after physiotherapy treatment.

Adductor longus

When resistance to femoral adduction develops, it becomes prominent and palpable at the junction with the pubic tubercle.

Pectineus

It is placed deep inside the femoral triangle and is felt to some extent outside the adductor longus tendon by applying resistance to flexion and adduction.

Gracillis

If a person sleeps and bends his knee 45 degrees, with resistance to thigh adduction and knee flexion, the muscle inside the thigh and its tendon inside the Semimembranosus muscle may be touched.

Adductor magnus

It has a muscle mass that can be felt and seen by resisting adduction of the thigh on the inside of the thigh and behind the adductor longus, but its tendon is located at the site of adhesion to the adductor tubercle in the depression between Vastus medialis and (ST) Semitendinosus. A tight rope is touched.

If the adductor muscles of the thigh are strong, the pants on the inside of the thigh will wear out. And if the muscles are paralyzed, the person walks loosely.

Hip muscles

Gluteus maximus

While a person is lying on his stomach or developing resistance to hip hyperextension, this muscle is identified. This muscle is also identified by pressing the buttocks together. The upper bouts featured two cutaways, for easier access to the higher frets, and the lower bouts featured two cutaways, for easier access to the higher frets.

Gluteus medius

These muscles, along with the gluteus minimus, are the strongest abductors of the hip joint. When standing, slightly below the iliac crest and on the outside of the gluteus maximus muscle, there is a depression called the gluteal depression. If there is resistance to abduction of the hip joint, this muscle can be felt in this depression. This muscle can also be better felt when the weight is on one leg. In this case, to prevent the pelvis from falling to the opposite side, it contracts sharply.

Trendelenburg sign (gait)

Normally, when standing on one leg, the upper side of both iliac crests is on the same level and the gluteus medius and minimus muscles prevent pelvic prolapse. However, in case of paralysis or weakness of the mentioned muscles or congenital dislocation of the hip joint (Congenital dislocation of the hip joint) or increase of the angle between the neck and the body of the thigh (Coax valga), the two iliac crest will not be on the same level. If the medius and minimus are paralyzed, the iliac crest will be placed on the same foot above the foot held high. If the muscles on the right side are paralyzed, the person bends to the right side while walking or grabs his bag or sack on the right side to make it easier to walk.

Hamstring muscles

Biceps femoris

By applying resistance to the knee flexion, it can be touched on the outside of the back of the thigh and its tendon can be seen as it moves towards the head of the fibula. This muscle forms the upper outer side of the popliteal fossa.

Semitendinosus

Its muscular part is located inside the long head of the Biceps femoris behind the thigh, and its tendon can be felt and seen by applying resistance to the knee flexion. This tendon is more prominent than other tendons inside and behind the thigh and is easily seen.

Semimembranosus

Although this muscle is thicker than the previous muscle, it is not easily touched. At the bottom, a large part of it is covered by Semitendinosus and at the top by Adductor magnus. Its tendon may be felt at the bottom on either side of the Semitendinosus tendon. The last two muscles form the inner and upper sides of the popliteal cavity.

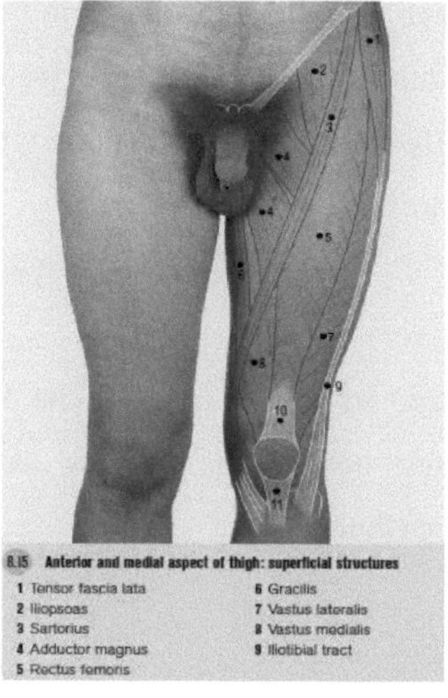

Figure 59. Superficial anatomy and surgery of the anterior thigh muscles

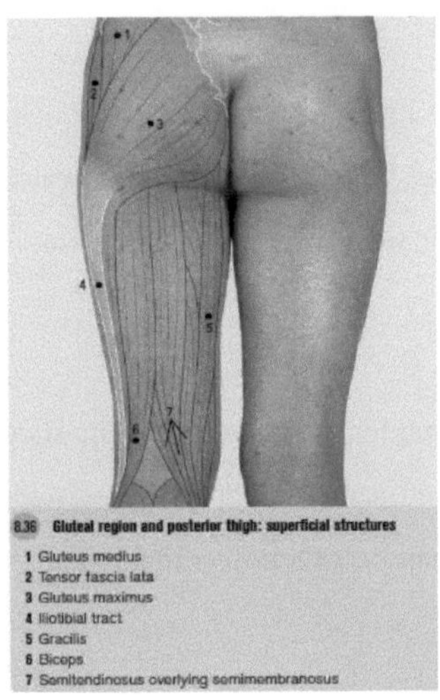

Figure 60. Superficial anatomy and surgery of the muscles behind the thigh

Muscles in front of leg

Tibialis anterior

The muscular part is immediately felt on the outside of the anterior side of the Tibia. Its tendon can be felt and seen in front of the ankle, in front of and outside the inner ankle, and inside the Extensor hallucis longus tendon. Resist Inversion and Dorsiflexion to better identify this muscle and tendon while the Interphalangeal and Metatarsophalangeal joints are bent.

Extensor hallucis longus

The muscular part is covered by the muscles of the front leg, but its tendon is immediately visible and felt outside the Tibialis anterior tendon by resisting Hyperextension of the big toe (thumb).

Extensor digitorum longus

The muscular part of the leg can be felt outside the anterior tibialis. Its tendon part in the ankle can be seen and touched by resisting the extension of the toes and Eversion on the outside of the Extensor hallucis longus tendon. Between the tendon of the last two muscles, the arteries and nerves of the Anterior tibialis pass. This muscle is eventually divided into 4 tendons for the last four fingers, and the tendon of each finger can be followed and touched to the end.

Proneus tertius

Extensor digitorum longus separates as a small tendon from the outside and goes to the surface behind the base of the fifth metatarsus and is palpable.

Muscles outside the leg and back of the leg

Proneus longus

With resistance to Eversion and Plantar flexion, it can be felt behind the external ankle and below the Proneal trochlea. The ventricular portion of Proneus longus may also be felt below the Fibula head.

Proneus brevis

With resistance to Eversion and Plantar flexion, the foot can be touched behind the external ankle and above the Proneal trochlea up to the base of the fifth metatarsus. This tendon is more specific than Proneus longus. It is located above the external ankle in front of the Proneus longus tendon.

Extensor digitorum brevis

By applying resistance to hyprextension of the metatarsophalangeal and interphalangeal joints of the fingers, the muscle mass in the front of the external ankle becomes well defined and palpable.

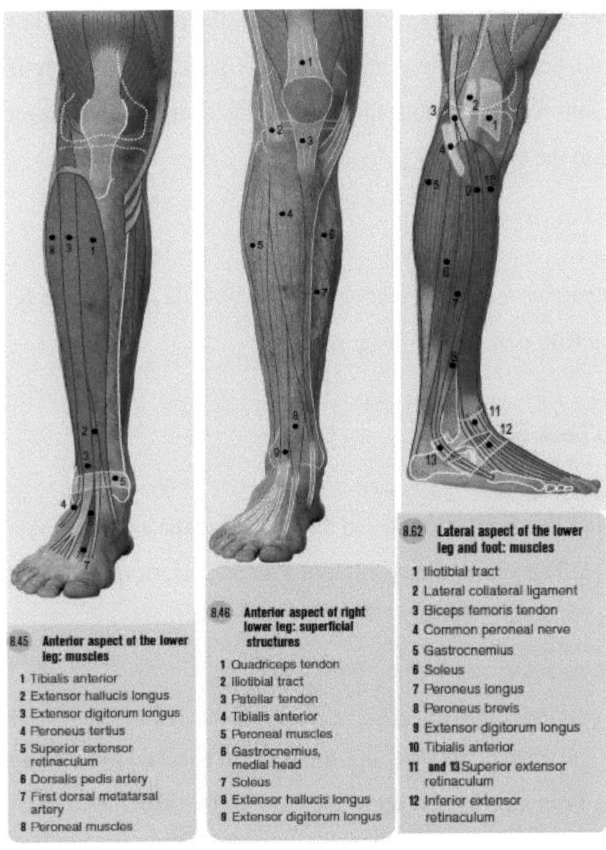

Figure 61. Anterior and lateral view of the calf muscles

Muscles of the back of the leg and sole of the foot

Triceps surae

It has three heads:

Gastrocnemius

The muscular protrusion forms the upper back of the upper leg, and with resistance to plantar flexion, both ends of the muscle are clearly visible and palpable. Walking, running and spinning are also seen when getting up on your toes.

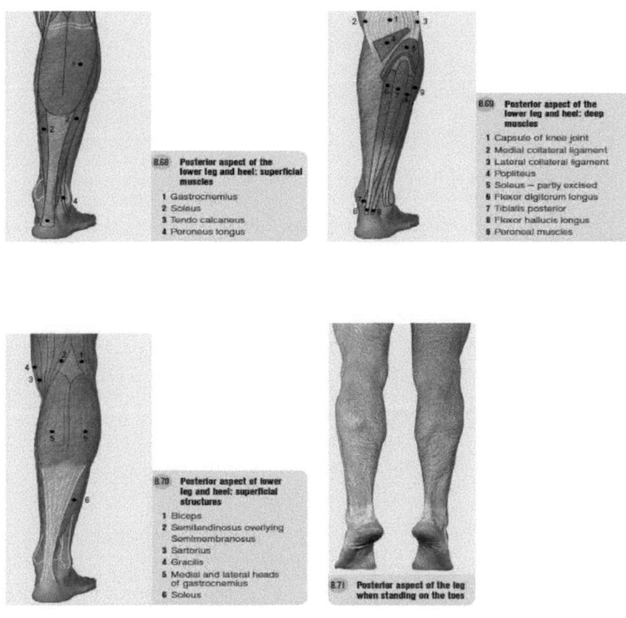

Figure 62. Posterior view of the calf muscles

Soleus

It is mainly covered by the Gastrocnemius muscle, but can be felt and seen in the lower part of the leg on either side of the muscle. To view this muscle, one must bend the knee and resist plantar flexion. These three parts of the muscle together form the strongest body tendon or Achilles tendon (Calcaneal or Achilles tendon) which is palpable and visible and is used as a good sign in superficial anatomy. Although this tendon is strong, it can rupture in athletes such as tennis players.

Tibialis posterior

With resistance to inversion and plantar flexion, the muscle tendon can be felt and seen above and below and behind the inner ankle.

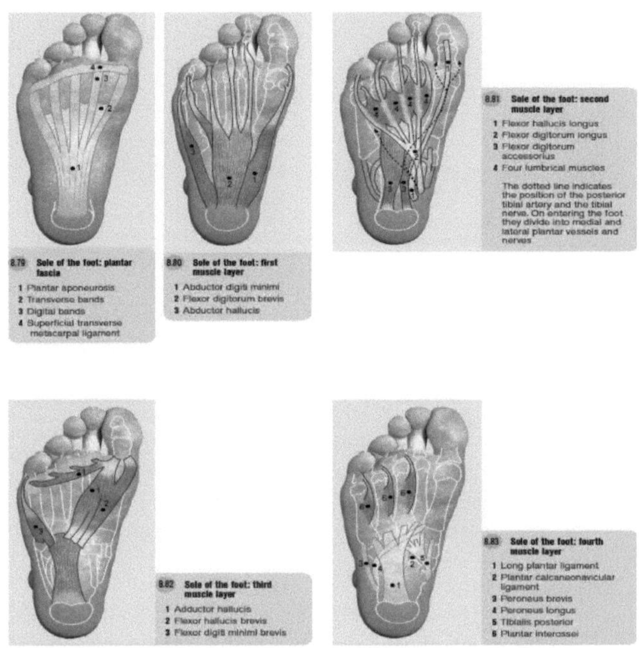

Figure 63. Superficial anatomy of the soleus muscles

Flexor digitorum longus

When the metatarsophalangeal and interphalangeal joints bend, the tendon is immediately palpable below the tibialis posterior tendon behind the medial ankle.

Flexor hallucis longus

The pulse of the posterior tibial artery is felt below and behind the Flexor digitorum longus tendon, and with flexion of the metatarsophalangeal and interphalangeal joints, the first finger can touch the tendon of this muscle immediately behind the pulse of the artery.

Abductor hallucis

If you resist pushing the distal ligament away from the big toe, you may touch this muscle on the inside of the foot.

Retinaculum and synovial sheaths around the ankle joint

The three leg muscle groups pass through the three sides of the ankle and are controlled by the retinaculum, which is the thickened fascia.

Flexor retinaculum

It is about 2.5 cm wide and extends from the inner ankle to the inner surface of the heel.

Peroneal retinaculum

It extends from the external ankle to the heel and has two upper and lower parts, the lower of which connects to the Inferior extensor retinaculum.

Extensor retinaculum

It has two parts:

Superior

It is at the top of the ankle joint and connects the bones of the fibula and tibia.

Inferior

It is Y-shaped, the stem originating from the heel and extending to the peroneal retinaculum. Its upper branch attaches to the inner ankle and its lower branch to the sole of the foot.

Synovial sheaths

Each tendon has its own synovial sheath, with the exception of the Peroneus tertius and Extensor digitorum longus tendons, which share a common synovial sheath.

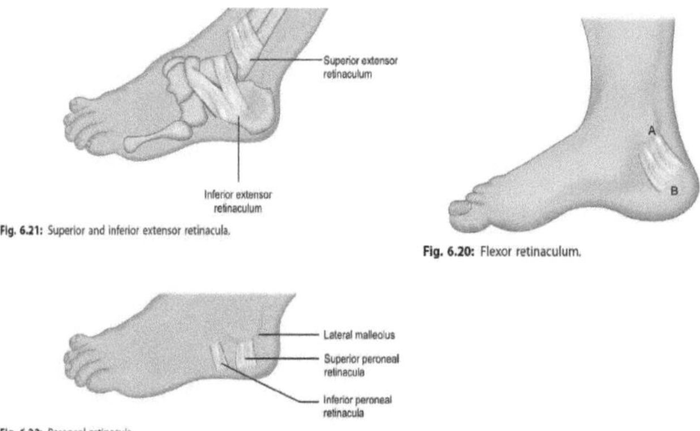

Figure 64. Lateral ankle ligaments

Areas and spaces of lower limbs

Inguinal (Poupart's) ligament

It is located between ASIS and the Pubic tubercle. At the bottom and outside of it is the inguinal fold. This ligament may be felt as a strong band inside the crease.

Inguinal fold

It is formed by bending the thigh and is oblique and is located 2 cm inside the inguinal ligament and 3-4 cm lower on the outside.

Femoral or Scarpa's triangle

It is bounded by the inguinal ligament above, the Sartarius on the outside, and the adductor longus on the inside. It contains arteries, nerves, and thighs. It is clinically important. By abduction and flexion and rotating out of the thigh, the boundaries of this triangle are determined.

Midinguinal point

It is the midpoint between the ASIS and the Symphysis Pubis and is where the femoral artery passes. About 1.25 cm (half an inch) below this point, the femoral arterial pulse is easily taken, and just above this point is the deep ring of the inguinal canal.

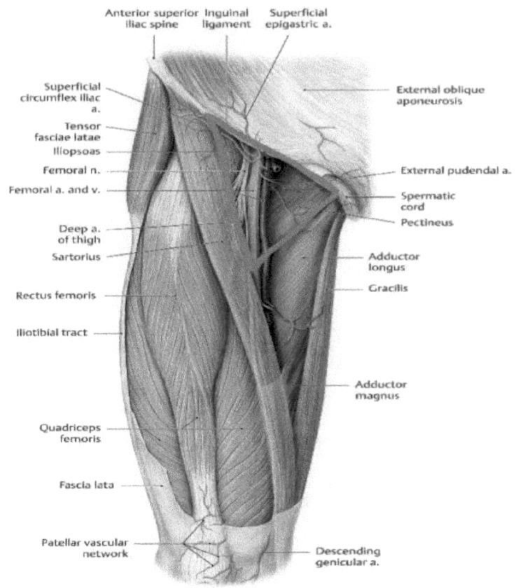

Figure 65. Superficial anatomy of the femoral triangle

Saphenous opening

It is an oval hole that pierces the Great Saphenous vein of the femoral fascia and flows into the femoral vein. The center of this hole is about 4 cm lower and 4 cm outside the pubic tubercle. Its small diameter is 2 and its large diameter is 2.5 cm long and it tends to the bottom and outside. This hole is located along the femoral canal, which is a common site of femoral hernia in women.

Femoral ring

It is located in the depth of the inguinal ligament and at a distance of one centimeter inside the mididing point and is the beginning of the femoral canal.

Midpoint of inguinal ligament

It is the midpoint between the ASIS and the pubic tubercle and is where the nerve conducts. This point is one centimeter outside the Midinguinal point.

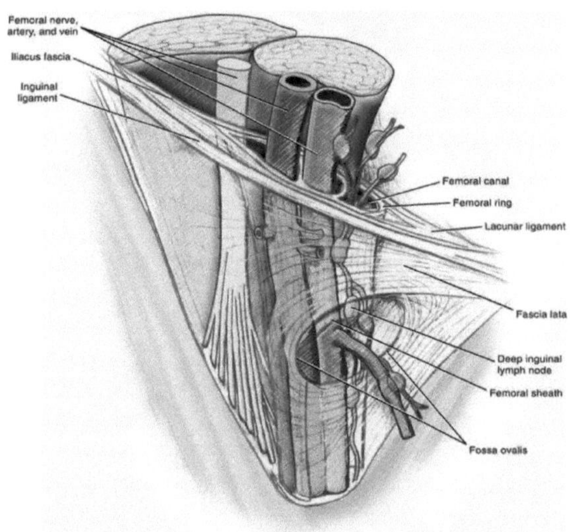

Figure 66. Superficial anatomy of the femoral triangle

Buttock or Gluteal region

It is an almost rectangular area whose sides are:

A) Inside, the natal cleft separates the two hips, starting at about the third sacral vertebra (S_3) and placing the Coccyx and the end of the sacrum at the base.

B) At the bottom, the gluteal fold on each side is a transverse line that separates the buttocks from the back of the thigh. This crease is caused by extension and is not formed by the lower side of the gluteus maximus muscle.

C) Above, Iliac crest. At the top and inside angle, there is a skin dimple, which is located in the area of this PSIS depression.

D) Outside, the line that descends perpendicular from ASIS.

In the standing position, the gluteal depression is located below the middle part of the iliac crest, where the Greater trochanter of the femur is palpable in the lower anterior part of the depression.

Adductor or Hunter's canal

It is located just below the apex of the thigh in the middle third of the thigh and is confined to the Vastus medialis on the outside and the Adductor muscles on the back and is covered by Sartorius on the front. This canal contains the femoral arteries and the saphenous nerve.

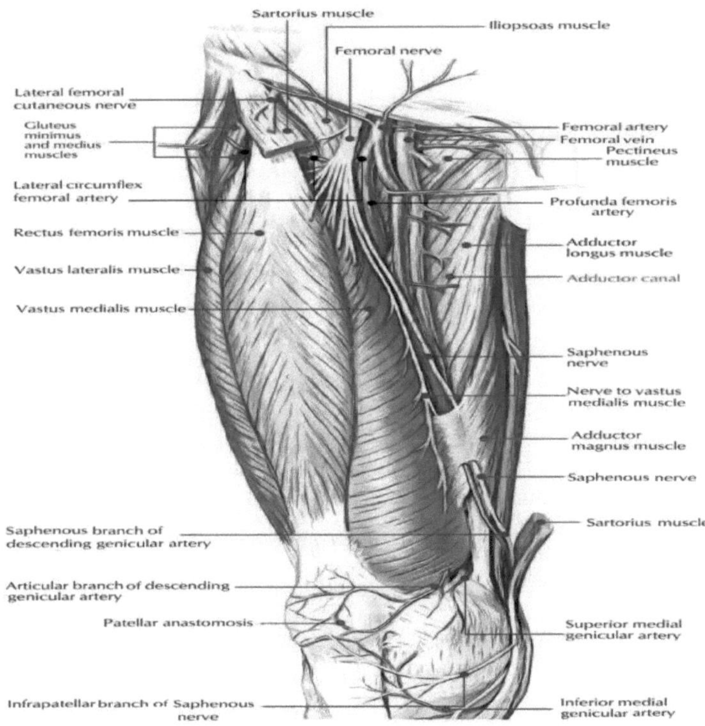

Figure 67. Anatomy of femoral and thigh triangle surgery

Depressions around the knee

Adductor depression

This depression is located between Vastus medialis and Semitendinosus. In the depth of this depression, the adductor tubercle and the adductor magnus tendon are palpable. This depression is best seen when the knees, ankles, and toes bend against resistance.

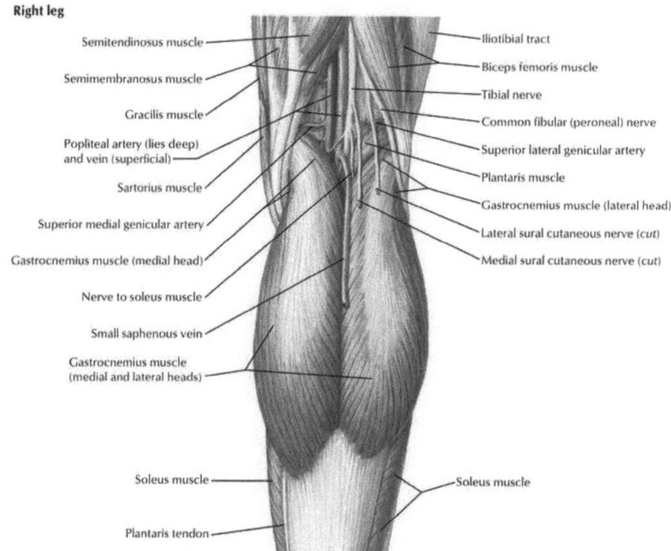

Figure 68. Anatomy of posterior femoral and posterior knee surgery

External depression

It forms between the Vastus lateralis and the Biceps femoris tendon. Immediately behind the Vastus lateralis is the iliotibial band, and when the person is lying down and the heel is slightly off the ground, the depression is marked by a groove with the knee slightly bent.

Popliteal fossa

The rhombus space is a shape located behind the knee. The upper sides are formed inside the Semitendinosus and Semimembranosus and outside the Biceps femoris, and the lower sides are formed by the inner and outer heads of the Gastrocnemius. Small saphenous vein and sural nerve pass on its surface. Tibial nerve, popliteal artery and popliteal vein are the contents of this cavity from surface to depth, respectively. The sides of this cavity are easily touched and seen (the artery is the deepest of all).

Nerves of the Lower Limb

The nerves of the lower extremities are deeper than the nerves of the upper extremities and are less accessible. However, the important nerve pathways of the lower extremities are given below.

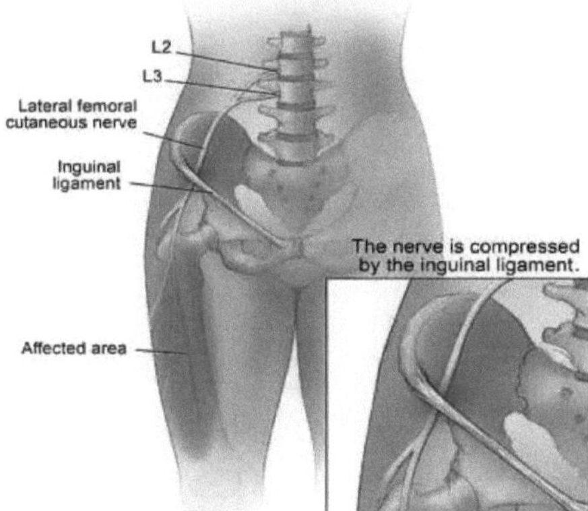

Figure 69. Lower limb nerves

Lateral cutaneous nerve of thigh

It is a direct branch of the lumbar network. Its path is linear in the abdomen, starting five centimeters outside the umbilicus and passing near the ASIS. At this point, it passes through the back or inside the inguinal ligament and then pierces the fascia, then divides into two branches, the front and the back, which innervate the thigh to the knee and participate in the neural network around the knee. When this nerve passes through the inguinal ligament, it may be under pressure and cause irritation and numbness of the outer thigh, which is called Meralgia Parasthetica. The nerve must be surgically removed from the ligament.

How to test the nerve: Stimulate the skin of the outer half of the thigh?

Nerve anesthesia site: near ASIS and Sartorius origin.

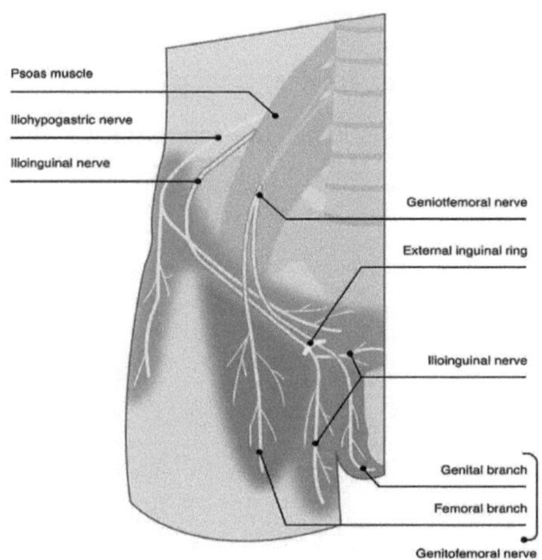

Figure 70. Lower limb nerves

Genitofemoral nerve

It exits the anterior surface of the Psoas major and is divided into two branches, Femoral and Genital. Its genital branch, after leaving the superficial inguinal ring, nerves the Cremaster muscle and the skin of the testicle and its adjacent area of the thigh. The femoral branch, along with the external iliac and femoral arteries, runs along the outer side behind the inguinal ligament and innervates the skin on the thigh triangle. To examine the first and second parts of the lumbar region (L_1-L_2) as well as to examine the descending of the testicle from the abdomen and its placement in the scrotum in the infant, stimulate the skin on the thigh triangle. In this case, the reflex contraction of the Cremaster muscle causes the testicles to rise. This test is called the Cremasteric reflex.

How to test a nerve: Stimulate the skin of the triangle?

Nerve anesthesia site: This nerve is deep but outside the pulse of the femoral artery and in the midpoint of the inguinal ligament anesthetic is injected. In this case, the nerve conduction is also anesthetized.

Obturator nerve

In the Intertubercular plane, the midline starts at a distance of 5 cm and descends vertically to reach the ASIS level. It then goes down and in and reaches 2.5 cm outside the pubic tubercle. This nerve is deep and gives nerves to the inside and top of the thigh.

How to test: Irritation of the skin inside and above the thigh.

Femoral nerve

To determine its direction, connect the following points:

A) The midpoint of the inguinal ligament or the width of a finger (1.5-5.5 cm) outside the pulse of the femoral artery.

B) 3-5 / 2 cm below point a. At this point, it is divided into muscle and skin branches, the most important branch of which is the saphenous nerve.

How to test a nerve?

1) Stimulation of the skin on the front of the thigh, inside the leg and on the inner ankle.

2) Patellar reflex or Knee jerk, which by hammering the Patellar ligament, in addition to nerve testing, the second, third and fourth parts of the lumbar (L_2-L_4) are also tested.

Saphenous nerve

The largest sensory branch is the neurotransmitter, which begins in the femoral triangle and is adjacent to the Sartorius muscle. At the top and back of the condyle, the inner thigh becomes superficial. If you draw a line from the back of the condyle inside the thigh to the front of the inner ankle, you have determined the path of this nerve in the leg. It travels along the Great Saphenous vein.

How to test the nerve: Stimulation of the skin inside the leg and on the inner ankle?

Nerve anesthesia site: In the middle point of the inguinal ligament.

Posterior cutaneous nerve of thigh

The sciatic nerve pathway is located but slightly inside it.

How to test the nerve: Irritation of the skin behind the thigh or the cavity behind the knee (Popliteal fossa).

Nerve anesthesia site: Slightly below the midpoint of the gluteal fold.

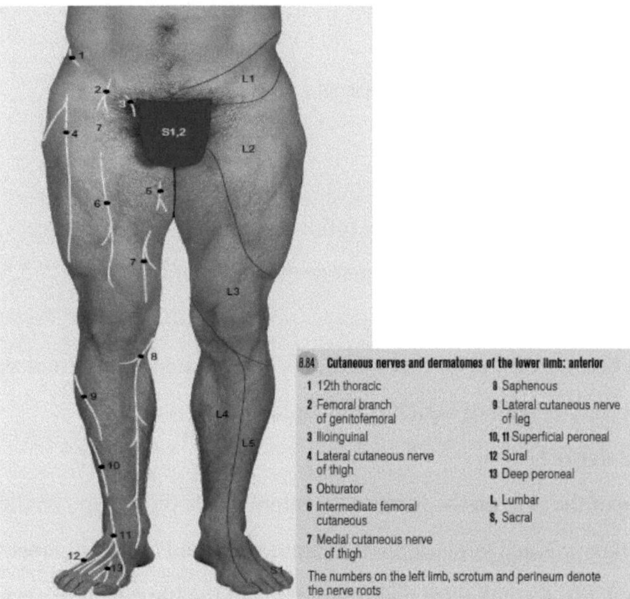

Figure 71. Lower limb nerves

Sciatic nerve

To determine its direction, connect the following points:

A) 2.5 cm outside the midpoint between PSIS and Ischial tuberosity.

B) Slightly inside the midpoint between the Greater trochanter and the Ischial tuberasity.

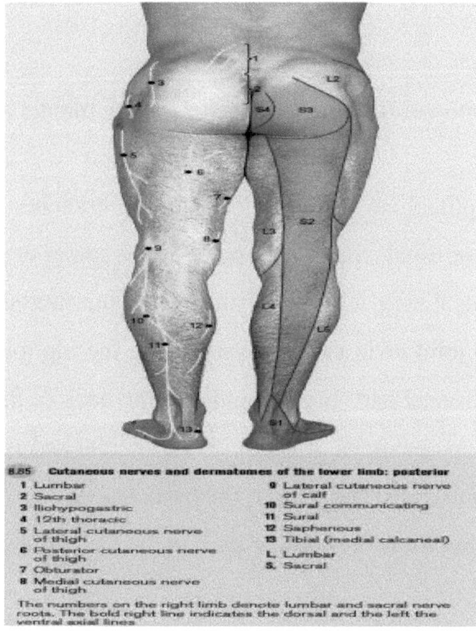

Figure 72. Lower limb nerves

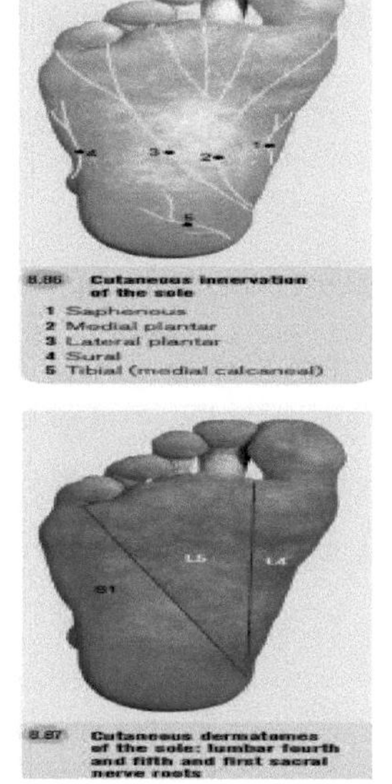

Figure 73. Plantar nerves

C) The apex of the popliteal fossa or the junction of the middle and lower third of the thigh.

At the apex of the popliteal cavity is divided into two branches, external or common peroneal and internal or tibial, which may occur in the upper or even in the pelvis. In the first part in the gluteal area, it may be damaged by intramuscular injections or back dislocation of the hip joint or in cases of surgery on the hip joint. Injections mainly affect the common peroneal part. In the middle of the back of the thigh, immediately after leaving the gluteus maximus, it becomes superficial and is covered only by the skin and fascia. In lumbar disc herniation, the branches of the sciatic nerve may also be pressed, causing symptoms of shooting pain in the back of the thigh and below the knee.

How to test a nerve: Stimulate the skin on the outside of the leg, sole and back of the foot, bend or straighten the ankle.

Anesthesia or electrical stimulation: Slightly below the midpoint of the gluteal fold.

Tibial nerve

Connect the following points:

A) The upper apex of the popliteal cavity or the junction of the lower third and upper two thirds behind the thigh.

B) The midpoint of the back of the leg at the level of the tibial tuberosity.

C) The midpoint between the heel and the inner ankle.

At this point (c) it is superficial and is located one centimeter behind the pulse of the posterior tibial artery.

How to test a nerve?

1) Irritation of the skin of the heel and back of the leg.

2) Plantar flexion.

3) Achille's tendon reflex.

Location of nerve anesthesia

1) Sciatica.

2) One centimeter behind the Posterior tibial pulse.

Sural nerve

Connect the following points

A) The lower angle of the popliteal cavity.

B) The distance between the outer ankle and the heel. It is accompanied by a small saphenous vein.

How to test the nerve: Stimulate the skin of the lower back and the back of the leg and the skin on the outside of the foot.

Location of nerve anesthesia

1) The lower apex of the popliteal cavity

2) In the distance between the outer ankle and the heel. In both places care must be taken that the needle does not enter the small saphenous vein.

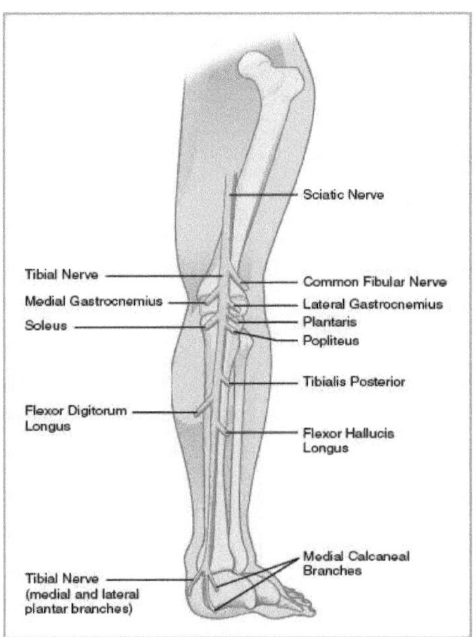

Figure 74. Leg nerves

Common peroneal nerve

Connect the following points

A) The upper apex of the popliteal cavity and the junction of the lower third and upper two thirds of the back of the thigh.

B) Fibula neck (about one centimeter below the apex of the Fibula). In this path, the nerve is located on the inner side of the Biceps femoris tendon and is about 4 cm below the apex of the fibula under the skin and can be touched. This nerve may be damaged in hip dislocation, hip injections, Fibula neck fractures, casts, and heel spurs due to improper use of splints, in which the ankle falls (Foot) drop). When walking, a person's fingertips are pulled to the ground, in addition to turning inward and forming a plantar flexion, creating a condition called Equinovarus.

How to test a nerve?

1) Irritation of the skin of the middle part of the back of the foot

2) Perform Dorsi flexion operation

3) Perform foot Eversion

Location of anesthesia or electrical stimulation of the nerve: Fibula neck.

Deep peroneal nerve

Connect the following points:

A) On the neck of the Fibula

B) 5 cm below the point between the Fibula head and the tibial tuberosity

C) The midpoint between the two ankles

D) The first space between the fingers that becomes superficial at this point.

From point B onwards, it is located on the outside of the anterior tibial artery.

How to test a nerve?

1) Stimulate the skin of the first space between the toes on the back of the foot.

2) Perform Dorsiflexion

Location of electrical stimulation of the foot Nerve anesthesia: Fibula neck

Superficial peroneal nerve

Connect the following points

A) Fibula neck

B) On the anterior side of Peroneus longus between the middle and lower third of the leg. At point b, the fascia is perforated and becomes superficial.

How to test a nerve?

1) Irritation of the skin on the back of the foot, except for the first space behind the foot.

2) Perform the Eversion operation.

Location of electrical stimulation or nerve anesthesia: Fibula neck

Medial plantar nerve

Connect the following points

A) The midpoint between the inner side of the Achilles tendon and the dorsal side of the inner ankle.

B) Tuberosity of the navicular, in the direction of the gap between the first and second toe in the sole of the foot.

How to test a nerve: Stimulate the skin 3.5 of the inner toe?

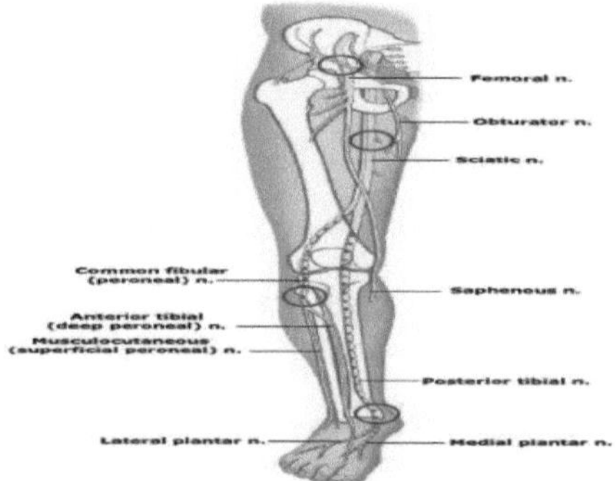

Figure 75. Leg nerves

Lateral plantar nerve

Connect the following points

A) The midpoint between the dorsal side of the inner ankle and the inner side of the Achilles tendon.

B) 2.5 cm inside the Tuberosiby fifth metatarsus in the sole of the foot.

C) The first space between the metatarsals in the sole of the foot. The distance between points B and C shows the path of the deep branch of the said nerve.

How to test the nerve: Stimulate the skin 1.5 external toes in the sole of the foot?

Nervous skin of the lower extremities

Hip area: Up and outside by Subcostal and Iliohypogastric nerves, inside by dorsal branches of lower lumbar and sacral nerves, below by Posterior cutaneous nerve of thigh.

Back of the thigh and Popliteal cavity: by the Posterior cutaneous nerve of the thigh.

External thigh: by Lateral cutaneous nerve of thigh.

Inside the thigh: from top to bottom by the Ilioinguinal, Obturator and Femoral nerves.

Anterior thigh: by the Medial and Intermediate branches of the cutaneous nerves of the thigh from the femoral nerve.

Inside the leg: On the inner ankle and the inner side of the foot by the saphenous nerve.

Outer leg: Above by the Lateral cutaneous nerve of the calf and at the bottom of the leg and back of the foot except the first space by the Superficial peroneal nerve.
The first space between the toes on the back of the foot by the Deep peroneal nerve.
The back of the leg and the outside of the foot by the Sural nerve.
Heel by Tibial nerve.
3.5 inner toes and the opposite skin from the sole of the foot except the heel by the medial plantar nerve and 1.5 outer toes and the opposite skin from the sole of the foot except the heel from the lateral plantar.

Dermatomes of Lower limb: Dermatomes of the lower limb are not simply upper limb due to fetal rotations.

Divide the front of the thigh into three parts from top to bottom. The upper area below the groin is innervated by the first lumbar spinal cord (L_1) and the skin on the knee by (L_3) and the middle area between the two by (L_2).

In the leg: Anteromedial part and inner ankle by (L_4), Anterolateral part and big toe (first) by (L_5).
Little (fifth) toe by S_1.

Upper back and popliteal cavity and back of thigh: by S_2.

Gluteal fold skin: inside by S_3 and around the anus by S_4.

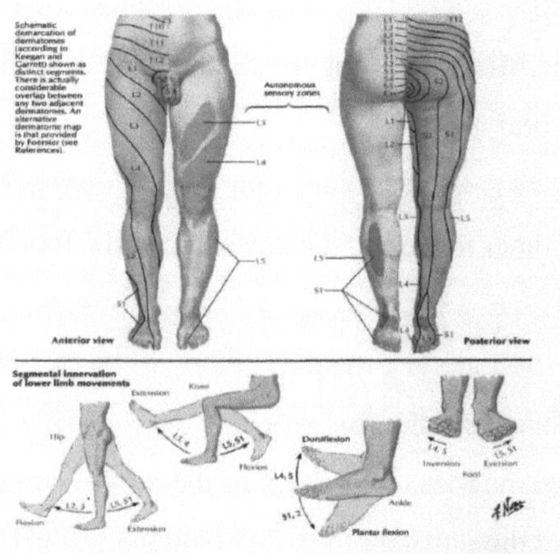

Figure 76. Dermatomes and lower limb movements

Intramuscular injections in the lower extremities

Lower limb injections are mainly in the buttocks and outside the thighs.

1) Valves under two years due to insufficient growth of the buttocks and the possibility of damage to the sciatic nerve, injection is done in the outer third of the middle thigh.

2) In the area below the Greater trochanter outside the thigh, which is a good place for diabetics to inject themselves, like injecting insulin.

3) Buttock region (Gluteal region) is the usual area for intramuscular injections, but in this area there is an injection into the sciatic nerve or nerves and arteries of this area and even sciatica. To determine the injection site, choose one of the following methods:
A) The upper and outer quarter of the gluteal region.
B) Place the index finger on the ASIS and the middle finger on the iliac crest. The space between these two fingers is a good place to inject (below the iliac crest behind the ASIS).
C) The front of the line that connects the PSIS and the Greater trochanter.

Arteries of lower limb

Superior gluteal artery

At the junction, the middle and upper third of the line connecting the PSIS to the Greater trochanter enters the hip area.

Inferior gluteal artery

About two centimeters outside the center of the line that connects the PSIS enters the hip area.

Femoral artery

To determine the surface path of the artery, connect the following points:
A) Midinguinal point in the continuation of the external iliac artery.
B) The connection of the lower and middle third of the line that connects point A to the adductor tubercle.
The upper half of the artery is in the femoral triangle and the lower half is inside the adductor canal. In the femoral triangle, the femoral nerve is located outside it and the femoral vein is located inside it. In this area, the pulse of the artery can be taken or the artery can be pressed to prevent bleeding. To make it easier to feel the pulse of the artery, it is better to place the relevant leg on the knee of the opposite leg. This artery is widely used to insert a tube into an artery (catheter), for angiography of arteries.

Profunda femoris artery

It is separated from the femoral artery 3.5 cm below the midpoint. First it goes down and out a little and then it goes down and in and reaches another point on the femoral artery at a distance of 10 cm from the Midinguinal point.

Popliteal artery

To determine the surface direction of this artery, connect the following points:

A) 2.5 cm inside the upper apex of the popliteal cavity (the junction of the upper two thirds and the lower third behind the thigh).

B) The middle part of the back of the knee (between the two condyles of the thigh).

C) The midpoint of the horizontal line at the back of the leg that is flush with the tibial tuberosity. At this point (c) it is divided into two end branches.

This is 5 cm below the upper side of the Tibia with the same level of Tibial tuberosity. If the knee is bent, the pulse of the popliteal artery can be felt behind the upper side of the tibia. At this point, the artery can be pressed to prevent bleeding. In addition, if necessary, you can close the blood pressure monitor on the thigh and place the phone on the pulse of the popliteal artery and measure blood pressure. It should be noted that lower limb blood pressure is usually higher than upper limb blood pressure.

Anterior tibial artery

If you connect the following points, the surface path of this artery is obtained:

A) The midpoint between the Fibula neck and the Tibial tuberosity.

B) The midpoint between the two ankles. In point B, the pulse of the mentioned artery can be touched. It is located here between the Extensor digitorum longus and Extensor hallucis longus tendons. The deep peroneal nerve is located outside this artery. Examination of the pulse of this artery and the dorsal artery is usually performed to examine the circulation of the lower extremities in diabetic and elderly patients.

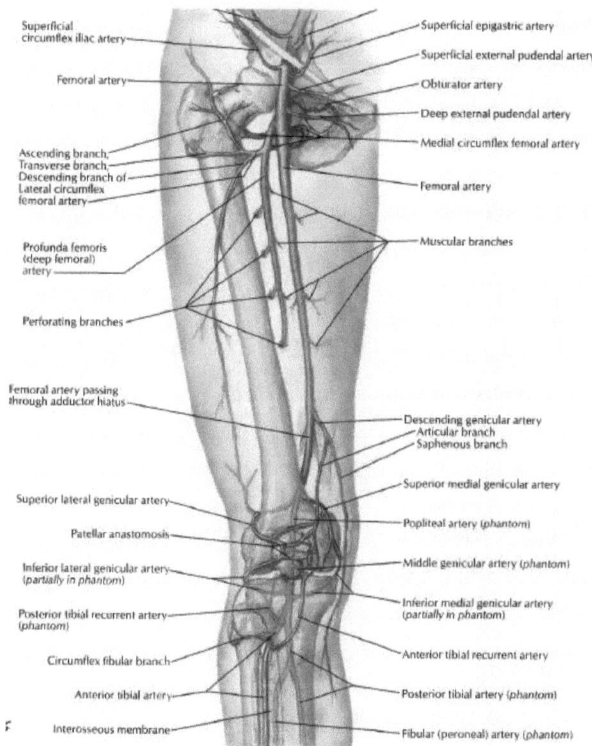

Figure 77. Blood vessels of the lower extremities

Dorsalis pedis artery

To identify the surface path, connect the following points

A) The midpoint between the ankles

B) Proximal end of the first space between the metatarsals

The pulse of the artery can be felt in this area outside the Extensor hallucis longus tendon, on the Cunieform bones, and outside the base of the first metatarsus. Sometimes this artery is used instead of the radial artery to insert a tube into a vein (catheter).

Posterior tibial artery

Connect the following points

A) The midpoint of the horizontal line drawn on the back of the leg is level with the tibial tuberosity.

B) The midpoint between the side of the Achilles tendon and the dorsal side of the inner ankle.

At point B, the pulse of the artery can be touched or the artery can be squeezed to prevent bleeding. In order to better feel the pulse of the artery, it is better for the foot to be in the position of Dorsiflextion and Eversion.

Peroneal artery

At the back of the leg, it separates from the beginning of the posterior tibial artery, on the outside, the posterior tibial artery descends approximately parallel to it and is deep.

Medial plantar artery

Connect the following points to get the surface path of the artery:

A) The midpoint between the inner side of the heel tendon (Achilles) and the dorsal side of the inner ankle.

B) Away from the navicular bone and in the direction of the gap between the first and second toe (about the middle of the heel and the base of the thumb).

Lateral plantar artery

By connecting the following points together, the surface path of this artery is determined.

A) The midpoint between the dorsal side of the inner ankle and the side inside the calcaneal tendon.

B) 2.5 cm inside the Tuberosity of the fifth metatarsus

Plantar arch

Lateral plantar and Dorsalis pedis arteries join. Its path is obtained by connecting the following points:

A) 2.5 cm inside the Tuberosity of the fifth metatarsus.

B) The rule of the first space between the metatarsals.

The path of this artery is slightly convex forward.

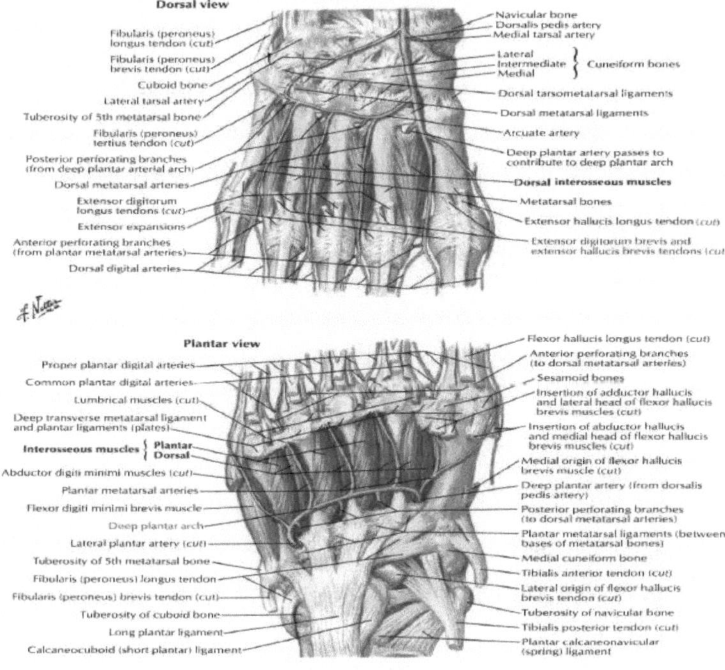

Figure 78. Ligaments and nerves of the sole of the foot

Veins of the lower limb

Lower extremity veins are clinically important because they are used for injections. Also, due to the fact that the veins of the lower extremities carry blood to the heart in the opposite direction of gravity, blood stasis may occur in the deep veins, especially after prolonged immobility, such as obstruction of surgery and long-term hospitalization takes place. Blood stasis may cause a thrombosis. Not only does the clot block the circulation in the vein, but the clot may be removed from the vein and enter the pulmonary or general arterial circulation, blocking a blood vessel and causing very severe pulmonary and sweat complications and even death.

Therefore, it is recommended that patients do not stay in bed for long periods of time and that after surgery or illnesses in which the patient is unable to walk, the patient's foot be actively moved by the patient or passively by others (such as nurses and physiotherapists). Avoid deadly complication.

Varicose veins are also very important for varicose veins. Blood is normally drained from the superficial veins by communicating veins into the deep veins. These communication veins have valves that control blood flow through the superficial veins to the deep veins. If the pressure in the deep veins increases (for example, due to excessive standing or mechanical obstruction in the vein), the valves of the communication veins will fail. As a result, blood returns to the superficial veins and the superficial veins dilate, which is called varicose (Varice = Varicose).

Prominent veins under the skin come in contact with clothing and may cause sores, bleeding and pain. Communication veins are usually closed for treatment.

The path of the deep veins is similar to that of the arteries, but the path of the superficial veins is as follows:

Dorsal venous arch or network: From the space between the metatarsals, the veins begin, where these veins join together to form the dorsal arch.

Small or short saphenous vein: Starts from the outside of the dorsal arch of the back of the foot. It then travels from the distance between the external ventricle and the Achilles tendon and enters the popliteal vein after piercing the deep fascia in the middle of the popliteal cavity. This vein accompanies the Sural Nerve.

Great saphenous vein: The tallest vein in the body. It starts from the inside of the venous arch of the back of the foot. Then it passes at a distance of 2.5 cm in front of the inner ankle of the foot. Following the path of the inner surface of the Tibia, it passes behind the inner condyles of the Tibia and Femor and is located behind the saphenous nerve. At the knee, it is about the width of a palm (10 cm) behind the inner side of the patella. In the thigh, the Sartorius muscle travels along the path and enters the femoral vein at the end in the saphenous opening.

This vein receives the superficial external pudendal veins, the superficial epigastric vein, and the superficial circumflex iliac. Specifically connect the following points to determine the surface path of this vein:

A) 2.5 cm in front of the inner ankle

B) Behind the condyle of the Tibia

C) Adductor tubercle

D) Saphenous opening

This vein accompanies the saphenous nerve for much of its path. This vein is used in the inner ankle area for Cutduwn. The saphenous veins are used to transplant blood vessels, for example in the heart (Coronary bypass).

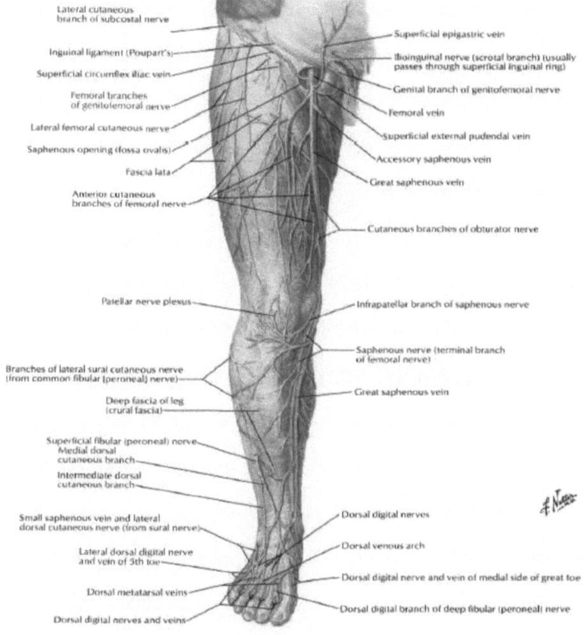

Figure 79. Lower limb veins

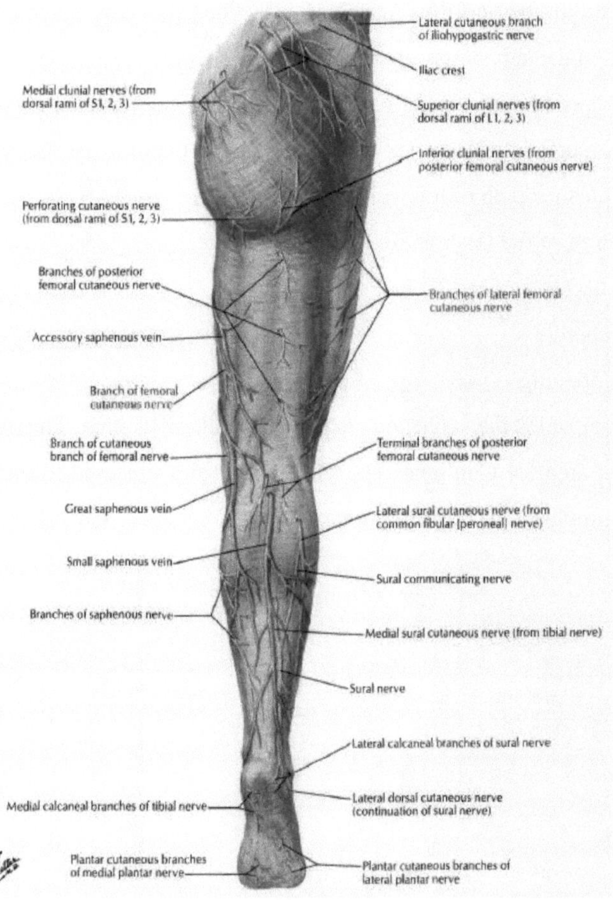

Figure 80. Lower limb veins

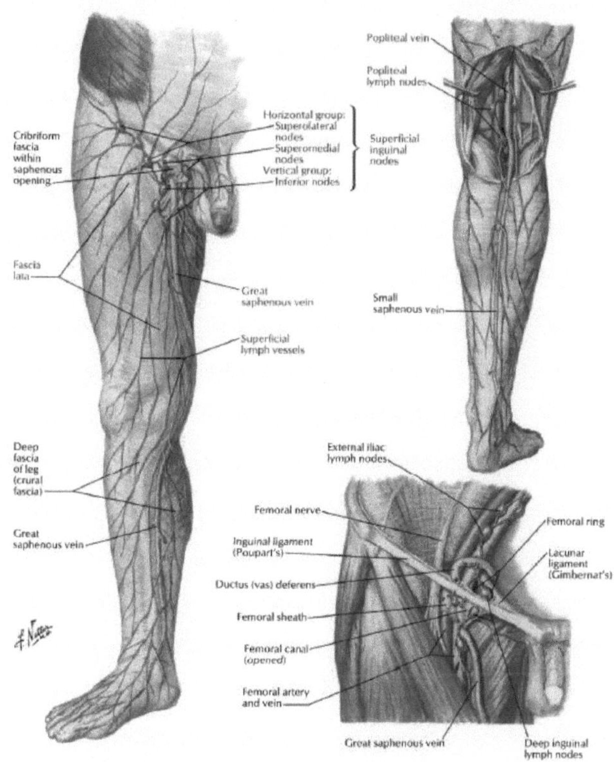

Figure 81. Lower limb veins

Lymph of the lower limb

By default, deep lymphatics follow the path of arteries and superficial lymphatics follow the path of superficial veins. The main drainage of lymph in the foot starts from the back of the foot. Therefore, it follows the path of small and large saphenous veins. The lymph from the outside of the foot and the back of the leg enters the popliteal lymph nodes and from here they enter the deep inguinal lymph nodes in the groin area. The lymph on the inside of the foot and the large saphenous vein route drain directly into the superficial inguinal lymph nodes of the groin. These nodes also receive the lymph between the perineum and the lower abdomen. These lymph nodes in the normal state may also be palpable. Pain and swelling in these nodes may indicate infection or malignancy in any part of the lymphatic drainage pathway.

References

1. Superficial anatomy of halim
2. Anatomy of Surgery Greys
3. Anatomy of Snell Surgery
4. Anatomy of Superficiality and Snell

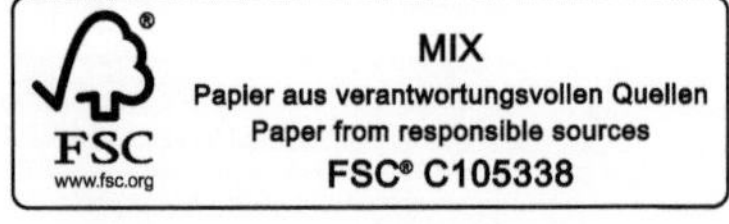

Printed by Books on Demand GmbH, Norderstedt / Germany